THE BIRTH OF THE TEXAS MEDICAL CENTER

NUMBER FIFTEEN:

Kenneth E. Montague Series in Oil and Business History

JOSEPH A. PRATT, GENERAL EDITOR

The Birth of the
Texas Medical Center

A PERSONAL ACCOUNT

By FREDERICK C. ELLIOTT

Edited with an Introduction by
WILLIAM HENRY KELLAR

Foreword by
RICHARD E. WAINERDI

TEXAS A&M UNIVERSITY PRESS
College Station

Library of Congress Cataloging-in-Publication Data

Elliott, Frederick C.
    The Birth of the Texas Medical Center : a personal account / by
    Frederick C. Elliott ; edited, with an introduction by William
    Henry Kellar.
        p. cm. — (Kenneth E. Montague series in oil and business
        history ; no. 15)
    Includes bibliographical references and index.
    ISBN 1-58544-333-6 (cloth : alk. paper)
    1. Elliott, Frederick C. 2. Texas Medical Center—History.
    3. Medical centers—Texas—Houston—History. 4. Health
    facilities—Texas—Houston—History. I. Kellar, William Henry,
    1952– II. Title. III. Series
    RA982.H62T494 2004
    362.11'09764'1411—dc22

                                              2004004494

For
the men and women
of the
Texas Medical Center

CONTENTS

LIST OF ILLUSTRATIONS   ix
FOREWORD, BY RICHARD E. WAINERDI   xi
EDITOR'S PREFACE   xv
INTRODUCTION   3

CHAPTER 1
The Long Road to Houston   21

CHAPTER 2
Texas Dentistry, Public Health, and the Texas Dental College   37

CHAPTER 3
Politics, Public Health, and
the Origins of the Texas Medical Center   61

CHAPTER 4
Building a Medical Center: The First Institutions, 1946–48   89

CHAPTER 5
Working Together: Public Funds and Private Philanthropy   109

CHAPTER 6
A New Era: Executive Director of the Texas Medical Center   125

CHAPTER 7
Making History: The Growth of the Texas Medical Center, 1956–59   153

CHAPTER 8
Expansion, Innovation, and Retirement, 1960–63   179

EPILOGUE   199
NOTES   209
A NOTE ON SOURCES   221
INDEX   223

ILLUSTRATIONS

Frederick Chesley Elliott, age three   23

Young Elliott with father and brother   25

Elliott's drugstore   28

Elliott as dean of the Texas Dental College   36

Texas Dental College   43

Technical Science Laboratory   44

Science Laboratory   45

Dental Clinic   46

Memorial Center for Health Education, architect's drawing   62

Memorial Center for Health Education, plaster model   64

Elliott as dean of Texas Dental College   65

Dedicatory dinner for Texas Medical Center   90

Elliott with Dr. Homer P. Rainey   94

Baylor College of Medicine's Cullen Building   101

M. D. Anderson Hospital for Cancer Research   122

Texas Medical Center construction   126

Ann Elliott and Fred Elliott   140

University of Texas Dental Branch   157

Elliott "working the crowd"   169

Elliott, Dr. R. Lee Clark, and Col. William B. Bates   195

Texas Medical Center, 2002   197

Ann Elliott and Fred Elliott, 1986   205

Dr. Frederick C. Elliott, 1986   206

FOREWORD

WHEN WILLIAM H. KELLAR asked me if I would write the foreword to his latest book, *The Birth of the Texas Medical Center: A Personal Account,* I responded positively and promptly. Frederick C. Elliott's career paralleled the early years of the Texas Medical Center, and he set a standard of excellence and integrity that has been a mark for all who followed.

William H. Kellar is an ideal choice among those who might have considered editing Dr. Elliott's papers and reordering them into a readable, cogent account of his life. In the early stages of his career as a historian, Kellar's education at Kent State University in Ohio and then at the University of Houston helped shape his ability to view modern higher education with the influences of an urban American setting. He can well understand the challenges Dr. Elliott and his colleagues faced when they sought to develop new and existing small schools and hospitals into major world-class institutions, capable of providing excellent health care, professional training, and education and related research.

Areas of teaching and research for Dr. Kellar include business and social history, medical history, and public history. His scholarship has already produced a number of books, including one on an outstanding Houston attorney's contribution to public life, an account of how the business of petrochemical technology enhanced Houston's international image, a serious study of the desegregation of Houston's primary and secondary school system, and an in-depth account of one of Houston's major private medical practices. All have been well received.

In choosing to work with the Elliott papers, Dr. Kellar selected a man who, during his lifetime, was well-known as a pharmacist, dentist, educator, administrator, and proponent of improved public health. Only a few people in Houston today enjoy the public acclaim and respect that was accorded Dr. Elliott during his career.

During the 1930s, Dr. Elliott was the highest-level health educator in Houston. He became a passionate advocate for improved public health and served on a variety of boards and health committees, including the Red Cross, Infantile Paralysis Foundation, the Houston Board of Health (of which he was president 1938–41), the Texas State Board of Health, and the Houston Chamber of Commerce Health Committee. All of this from a man who arrived on the Houston scene in 1932 to become the dean of the struggling Texas Dental College. Over the next decade, Elliott brought that school back from the brink of failure and engineered the assimilation of the Texas Dental College into the University of Texas System. He continued to serve as dean of the University of Texas Dental Branch until his appointment as executive director of the Texas Medical Center in 1952—yet another example of his quiet and efficient manner to achieve what few others would even attempt.

Dr. Elliott was one of the nine signers of the original charter establishing the Texas Medical Center in 1945, and even in that there is a touch of his humility and quiet sense of humor. In an account recalled by others who were present at the time, Dr. Elliott was actually the first person to sign the charter. Dr. Ernst W. Bertner and Dr. Elliott were good friends and they had worked on the charter's wording for some days, between doing all the other things they each needed to do. At the end, Dr. Bertner gave the final draft to Dr. Elliott to take it for one last review by attorney John H. Freeman. When Mr. Freeman finished looking at it, he turned to Dr. Elliott and asked him if he was satisfied with it. Dr. Elliott said yes, and Mr. Freeman said, "Then sign it." Thus, Dr. Elliott was the first signatory of the document to be presented to the Texas Secretary of State to form the incorporation of the new Texas Medical Center.

Dr. Bertner was named executive director of the center, and Dr. Elliott continued working behind the scenes to help the new organization. When Dr. Bertner died, Dr. Elliott assumed the post of executive director. He served in this capacity from 1952 onward for the next eleven years, providing steady, able leadership during a time of rapid development of the Texas Medical Center.

Dr. Elliott was a modest man, not a self-promoter, and he preferred, even during the years he was executive director, to work behind the scenes. Consequently, his contributions may not be as well-known as those of other Texas Medical Center founders. In 1970, however, he was given the Texas Medical Center Medallion in recognition of his contributions as one of the founders and principal leaders of the Texas Medical Center. Only a few medallions have been given during the nearly sixty-year history of the Texas Medical Center, but none was more deserved than the one given to Dr. Frederick C. Elliott.

William H. Kellar's editing of the Elliott papers and his scholarly gathering of additional information to make a complete biography is also a fitting tribute to a man who not only had a vision of a medical city but also spent much of his life building it.

—RICHARD E. WAINERDI,
President, Chief Executive Officer,
and Chief Operating Officer,
Texas Medical Center

EDITOR'S PREFACE

WHILE I WAS CONDUCTING RESEARCH to write the history of Houston's Kelsey-Seybold Clinic, Dr. Mavis P. Kelsey mentioned that his old friend and one of the pioneers in the development of the Texas Medical Center, Frederick C. Elliott, D.D.S., had written a memoir manuscript that told the story of the early days of the Medical Center. Dr. Elliott served as dean of the Texas Dental College (later the University of Texas Dental Branch) for twenty years and as executive director of the Texas Medical Center for ten years. He wrote most of his manuscript in 1976 and intended to publish it as a book. However, the project languished, and Dr. Elliott died before any further action could be taken. Kelsey had read the manuscript and promised Ann Orr Elliott, Dr. Elliott's widow, that he would see about getting it published. Many years passed between Elliott's death and my conversation with Dr. Kelsey, and the manuscript project seemed to have been lost along the way. The idea sounded interesting to me, so I told Dr. Kelsey that I would attempt to find a copy and see what could be done about publishing it. Elizabeth White, director of the McGovern Historical Collections and Research Center in the Houston Academy of Medicine–Texas Medical Center Library, made available a typed hard copy, as well as diskettes of Elliott's work.

The manuscript provided an interesting look at the development of the Texas Medical Center and the University of Texas Dental School. However, Elliott's formal Victorian writing style needed considerable editing and some additional research to corroborate his recollections, as well as to provide historical background information. As I began conducting research and editing, I watched a 1973 videotaped interview of Dr. Elliott and tried to develop a sense of the man and the way he communicated his thoughts. I approached the task of editing with caution, taking care to keep the authenticity of Elliott's voice and yet to iron out excessive use of passive voice and some of his old-style conventions found throughout the text (such as not identifying first names, the formal use of "Mr." and "Mrs."). In addition,

I reorganized the text, deleted wandering passages that distracted from the main theme, and integrated an autobiographical essay that Dr. Elliott wrote early in 1986 into chapter 1 of his original manuscript.

Additional research included a careful examination of TMC-related papers in the McGovern Historical Collections of the HAM–TMC Library; conducting a series of about fifteen oral history interviews with key people in the Texas Medical Center; and a review of appropriate secondary source literature, newspaper articles, and clippings files in other Houston-area libraries.

Although some institutions predate it, the Texas Medical Center has existed as a formal entity for nearly sixty years, yet the secondary literature about this medical complex is somewhat limited. Several histories have been written about individual institutions in the Medical Center including *A History of Baylor University College of Medicine, 1900–1953*, by Walter H. Moursand, 1956; *The First Twenty Years of the University of Texas M. D. Anderson Hospital and Tumor Institute*, edited by Dr. R. W. Cumley and Joan McCay, 1964; *A Guide to the Texas Medical Center*, by Clyde W. Burleson and Suzy Williams Burleson, 1987; *The Methodist Hospital of Houston: Serving the World*, by Marilyn McAdams Sibley, 1989; *Memories: A History of The University of Texas Dental Branch at Houston*, by Dr. E. W. D'Anton, 1991; *The History of Surgery in Houston: Fifty-Year Anniversary of the Houston Surgical Society*, edited by Dr. Kenneth L. Mattox, 1998; *Conversation with a Medical School: The University of Texas-Houston Medical School, 1970–2000*, by Drs. Bryant Boutwell and John P. McGovern, 1999; *Twentieth-Century Doctor: House Calls to Space Medicine*, by Dr. Mavis P. Kelsey, Sr., 1999; *Kelsey-Seybold Clinic: A Legacy of Excellence in Health Care*, by William Henry Kellar and Vaishali J. Patel, 1999; *The Quest for Excellence: Baylor College of Medicine, 1900–2000*, by Ruth SoRelle, 2000; *The Good Old Days: Memoirs of Retired Harris County Physicians*, edited by Dr. George Alexander, 2001; and a series of books written by N. Don Macon and published by the Texas Medical Center including: *Mr. John H. Freeman and Friends: A Story of the Texas Medical Center and How it Began*, 1973; *South From Flower Mountain: A Conversation with William B. Bates*, 1975; *Clark and The Anderson: A Personal Profile*, 1976; and *Monroe Dunaway Anderson, His Legacy: A History of the Texas Medical Center, 50ᵗʰ Anniversary Edition*, 1994. New books being written presently include a history of the Texas Children's Hospital and an updated history of the University of Texas M. D. Anderson Cancer Center.

The final manuscript comprises ten chapters, including eight chapters of Dr. Elliott's text, along with an introduction and an epilogue written by myself. It should be noted that many of the institutions of the Texas Medical Center have changed names, and some have changed affiliations over the years. I have attempted to make note of these changes in the text. Also, I have moved some of Dr. Elliott's comments to a notes section at the end of the book and have added corroborating information to these notes, as well. The result is an inside look at the developmental years of the University of Texas Dental Branch and the Texas Medical Center through the eyes of one of the founding members. This book is an important addition to the existing body of knowledge about the development of the Texas Medical Center and to the evolution of health care in Houston during the twentieth century.

MANY PEOPLE PROVIDED ENCOURAGEMENT and assistance for this project, and I never could have completed it without their help. First and foremost, I want to thank Dr. Mavis P. Kelsey, Sr., for introducing me to this manuscript. I first met Dr. Kelsey in 1998 while writing a history of the Kelsey-Seybold Clinic, which he founded in 1949. Dr. Kelsey knew Frederick Elliott and many of the people who contributed to establishing the Texas Medical Center. In addition, he has written frequently about the history of medicine in Houston, including an autobiography, *Twentieth-Century Doctor: House Calls to Space Medicine,* and thus proved to be an invaluable source of information. We spent many pleasant hours talking about Frederick Elliott, the Texas Medical Center, and a host of other things, all of which helped me to gain an understanding of the times and the issues surrounding the creation of the Medical Center. Dr. Kelsey is a renowned physician and scholar, and I remain forever grateful for his support and his friendship.

In addition to Dr. Mavis P. Kelsey, several other luminaries of the Texas Medical Center graciously made time in their busy schedules to share their recollections of Dr. Elliott and the "early days." Dr. Denton A. Cooley talked about his first years in the Medical Center and at St. Luke's Episcopal Hospital. He also shared some wonderful personal stories about Frederick Elliott's long friendship with his family. Dr. William D. Seybold knew Frederick Elliott very well and actually interviewed him for an earlier Medical Center history project. Dr. Seybold graciously consented to an interview in which he shared his remembrances of Elliott and also of his own career at a number of institutions in the Texas Medical Center. Dr. Michael E. DeBakey talked about the early days at Baylor College of Medicine and the Methodist Hospital. Dr. Richard E. Wainerdi, president of the Texas Medical Center, shared his perspective on the people and institutions of the Texas Medical Center and also provided encouragement and support for this project. Mary Schiflett, vice president of public affairs for the Texas Medical Center, was exceedingly generous in sharing her recollections and wise counsel at key points during the project. She and her assistant, Tracy Murley, also provided a variety of helpful reports and information about the Medical Center. In addition, Dr. Chester R. Burns at the University of Texas Medical Branch at Galveston, Dr. John P. McGovern, Paul Gervais Bell, Thomas D. Anderson, and Searcy Bracewell generously made time in their busy schedules to share their recollections and observations about Frederick C. Elliott and the development of the Texas Medical Center. Late in the project, I had the good fortune to meet Dr. Leslie O. Fullerton, executive vice dean of the University of Texas Health Science Center at Houston Dental Branch. Dr. Fullerton was very supportive of the project and introduced me to Dr. E. W. "Danny" D'Anton. Dr. D'Anton, a retired professor from the Dental Branch and author of a history of the school, was well acquainted with Dr. Elliott. He generously provided rare photographs and shared personal anecdotes that proved to be invaluable contributions to this book. Finally, Dr. William G. Squires, Jr., Dr. Charles H. Oestreich, and Dr. Ralph Sagebiel of Texas Lutheran University graciously shared their recollections of Dr. Elliott and enabled me to discover a chapter of his life that was unknown to most Houstonians.

This project could not have been done without the support of the Houston Academy of Medicine–Texas Medical Center Library. First, I am grateful to have been the recipient of a research grant that enabled me to cover some of the expenses involved in the project, including travel, interviewing, transcribing, and photocopying. In addition to this financial support, the HAM–TMC Library has a wonderful collection of books, papers, audiotapes, videotapes, and artifacts relating to the history of medicine. Elizabeth Borst White, director of the John P. McGovern Historical Collections and Research Center at the Houston Academy of Medicine–Texas Medical Center Library was deeply involved in this project. Through her vast knowledge of the holdings in the HAM–TMC Library, Beth was able to offer suggestions and direction as I conducted my research. Dennis Moser, Pam Cornell, Kimberly Youngblood, and Sara Holland also helped in countless ways, both big and small, to unlock the doors to the many treasures in the library's collection. Sadly, the massive flooding from Tropical Storm Allison in the summer of 2001 destroyed many precious documents and artifacts in the McGovern Historical Collections. Still, I must salute the staff who worked valiantly under terrible conditions to save as much as possible. They continued their work and also provided assistance to me with great patience and good cheer.

Many people outside of the Houston medical community contributed to this project. Sonia Fadwa Richi reformatted, edited, and retyped most of the original manuscript so that it would be compatible with modern word processing software. The work was tedious, and without her efforts this project could not have moved forward. Ami Patel, my lead research assistant and photographer, worked diligently to help process documents and other information critical to the project. Researchers Ronnate Asirwatham and Jeanie Dang provided additional research help. Suzanne Mascola transcribed all of the interviews, including recordings of the Macon video interviews with many of the TMC founders. Paul Pendergraft, a journalist at KUHF radio in Houston, shared his informed perspective on the people and institutions of the Texas Medical Center. Kay Schlembach skillfully created the index. Also, I want to express my deepest gratitude to Vaishali Patel, my collaborator on a previous project, who graciously read and commented on several versions of this manuscript, and to Joseph A. Pratt, History Department Chair at the University of Houston, for his suggestions and insights related to this project.

The staff at Texas A&M University Press once again proved to be among the most professional and pleasant teams in the world of academic publishing. Finally, to my faithful staff at the University of Houston Scholars' Community program, my sincere thanks for their patience, understanding, and support during the sometimes stressful moments of trying to juggle too many projects at one time. And to the many others who remain anonymous, my heartfelt thanks for your support.

THE BIRTH OF THE TEXAS MEDICAL CENTER

INTRODUCTION

FREDERICK CHESLEY ELLIOTT'S LIFE spanned nearly a century, and, in his time, he was well known as a pharmacist, dentist, educator, administrator, and champion of public health. He served for twenty years as the dean of both the Texas Dental College and the University of Texas Dental Branch (now the University of Texas Health Science Center at Houston Dental Branch) and was the guiding force behind that institution's affiliation with the University of Texas. Elliott was a visionary and one of the pioneers of the Texas Medical Center. His efforts on behalf of the Medical Center and public health in Houston have left a legacy of service unparalleled in modern times. And yet today, nearly twenty years after his death in 1986, Frederick C. Elliott remains the most enigmatic figure among the founders of the Texas Medical Center. Elliott's legacy looms large but mostly silent in the place he loved so much. Why is this so? Who was this remarkable man, and why has his name all but disappeared from the pantheon of Medical Center founders?

Most traditional accounts about the origin of the Texas Medical Center begin with Monroe D. Anderson and the establishment of the M. D. Anderson Foundation in 1936. The central role of the Anderson Foundation in the development of the Texas Medical Center is clear and beyond dispute, but the originator of the idea for a medical center in Houston is less clear. This might be, as the evidence suggests, because several people had ideas about establishing some kind of comprehensive medical facility in the city. It is widely acknowledged that the charismatic Dr. Ernst William Bertner was the guiding force during the founding era of the Texas Medical Center. He began to envision a medical-educational complex shortly after he first arrived in Houston in 1913. Less well-known is the fact that Elliott was also among those community leaders who saw a need for improved public health services in Houston. As the dean of the only health-related institution of higher education in the city, Elliott felt a responsibility to speak out about this issue. In 1938, he became one of the first to envision and publicly advocate a combined central medical school and teaching hospital for Houston, which he called the Memorial Center for Health Education.[1]

Described by those who knew him as a modest, self-effacing person, Elliott endured the tribulations of his life with grace and dignity. He was generally content to be the man behind the scenes, while his more charismatic colleagues engaged in the public roles of building support for the Texas Medical Center. Although he is largely forgotten today, Elliott was well-known and highly respected by the business, political, and community leaders of his time. He was frequently recognized for his work as a superb dentist, an innovative educator, and as one of the founders of the Texas Medical Center. In April, 1941, the Houston Rotary Club proclaimed Elliott the "Man of the Month." In 1959, the Houston District Dental Society honored him as the "Dentist of the Century," and in 1960, he received a Gold Medal from the Pierre Fauchard Academy. The Fauchard Academy is an International Honor Dental Organization that was established in 1936 and named in honor of Pierre Fauchard, a French dentist who is recognized as the father of modern dentistry.

During his lifetime, Elliott received many additional awards and honors. On March 19, 1970, his contemporaries recognized his contributions to the University of Texas Dental Branch and to the Medical Center when the Texas Medical Center's board of directors held a luncheon to honor him and Col. William B. Bates "for their dedicated work and leadership." Both Dr. Elliott and Colonel Bates were presented the Texas Medical Center Medallion in recognition of their contributions as principal leaders "in the establishment, development, and continued progress of the Texas Medical Center."[2]

In the chapters that follow, Frederick C. Elliott provides a brief account of his life and how he ultimately became one of the founders and early leaders of the Texas Medical Center. His autobiography is not a complete historical account, but it is very useful because he tells the story of those early days from his unique perspective. As one of the major players during the formative years, Elliot's observations and recollections provide an invaluable resource for administrators, scholars, and the public at large who are interested in the early history of the Texas Medical Center.

Frederick C. "Fred" Elliott was born in Pittsburg, Kansas, on October 23, 1893. He developed a strong work ethic and a stoic manner during a childhood in which he lost his mother at the age of four and later contracted polio. After his mother died, he began helping out in his father's drugstore. He studied pharmacy and passed his board exam when he was just seventeen years old. After several attempts to run his own drugstore, he became weary of the long hours and decided upon a new career.

Elliott entered the Kansas City Dental College and received his degree in 1918. The dean recognized Elliott's ability to communicate and offered him a faculty appointment. With World War I drawing to a close, the future looked bright for Dr. Elliott and his bride of three years, the former Anna Bracket. The couple was expecting their first child and beginning to enjoy Elliott's steady income when tragedy struck once again. In November, 1918, both Anna and her premature baby died as a result of the flu epidemic that was sweeping the world. For the next ten years, Elliott found solace from his grief by focusing on his work and by writing poetry. During the spring of 1928, Elliott married Phrania Anna Orr (Ann) and accepted an appointment to the faculty of the University of Tennessee College of Dentistry in Memphis.

In 1932, Elliott agreed to accept an appointment as dean of the struggling Texas Dental College in Houston. He arrived in Houston on August 15, shortly after a major hurricane, to find a city inundated by rains and the dental school basement flooded. N. Don Macon, a film producer and author who interviewed many of the Texas Medical Center's founders, including Elliott, wrote that "Dr. and Mrs. Elliott found temporary living quarters in a tourist court on South Main Street, near the Texas Dental College at Fannin and Blodgett. It rained for a week. The streets overflowed, and water poured into the basement of the building. Students and teachers stripped themselves to the waist, removed their shoes and socks, and bailed out the dental school." This was Fred Elliott's welcome to his new home, but he was not discouraged. Although Houston's population barely touched 300,000 when Elliott first arrived in 1932, there was a vigor, a can-do spirit, in the community that was palpable. Elliott mentioned this frequently in his writings and believed that the potential for both the city and the Texas Dental College were limitless. As Don Macon wrote many years later, Fred Elliott "knew then and there that, come hell or more high water, he was going to make a go of this job."[3]

But making a go of his new job was not going to be easy. Dean Elliott was fighting a declining enrollment, financial difficulties, and the new trend by accrediting boards to deny accreditation to dental schools that did not have a university affiliation. Determined to save the school, Elliott carefully orchestrated a strategy to gain support for affiliating the dental college with a four-year university. He sought backing from the Houston business and medical communities and from the University of Texas Medical Branch at Galveston (UTMB).

At that time a local public school system, the Houston Independent School District, which administered a junior college, had been developing plans to turn the institution into a four-year university, to be called the University of Houston. Elliott met with school board members, including Col. William B. Bates, the board president, to convince them to include the dental school in their plans for the university. However, as Bates recalled years later, the board was not interested in an affiliation with the Texas Dental College. Dr. Ray K. Daily, a school board member, blocked the idea because the dental college seemed likely to become a financial burden on the school district. Elliott had met Colonel Bates months earlier, but his efforts to win the approval of the board members provided an opportunity for the two men to become better acquainted. Although he was disappointed by the school board's decision, Elliott's acquaintance and ensuing friendship with Bates would play an important part in the future of the dental college and the Texas Medical Center.[4]

Rebuffed by the local public school district and also by the University of Texas Medical Branch in Galveston, Elliott continued his campaign to raise the profile of the dental school. As dean of the Texas Dental College, the only medical institution of higher education in the city at the time, Fred Elliott was the highest-level health educator in Houston. In this capacity, Elliott spoke to various groups in the Houston community and around the country. He served on several boards and health committees including the Red Cross, Infantile Paralysis, the Houston Board of Health (serving as president 1938–41), the Texas State Board of Health (1941–43), and the Houston Chamber of Commerce Health Committee (1938–42). Fred Elliott became acquainted with many influential community and political leaders through his work on these local and state organizations. His interest in public health became a lifelong concern during these years and ultimately led to his role as one of the founders of the Texas Medical Center.[5]

A series of events during the 1930s proved to be crucial in paving the way for the development of the Texas Medical Center a decade later. Sometime in the mid-1930s, Elliott first met Dr. Ernst W. "Bill" Bertner through their work together on the Chamber of Commerce Health Committee. Bertner was a native Texan, born in Colorado City. He was a graduate of the University of Texas Medical Branch at Galveston and a World War I veteran. Bertner had been enticed to come to Houston by Jesse H. Jones, a successful businessman and community leader, who wanted the charismatic young physician to be the house doctor in his newly opened Rice Hotel. A lifelong friendship between Elliott and Bertner grew during their time together on the City Health Commission when they took on the city council in a losing effort to improve public health facilities. Elliott and Bertner became a formidable team as advocates for improved public health in Houston.

In June, 1936, a wealthy Houston businessman, Monroe D. Anderson, established the M. D. Anderson Foundation. Anderson had moved to Houston in 1907 to represent his cotton trading firm, Anderson, Clayton & Company, which was first established in Oklahoma City on August 1, 1904. The company prospered in Houston, and by the 1930s, Anderson and his remaining partners, Will Clayton and Lamar Fleming, had become quite wealthy. But there was a problem that the partners faced as they grew older. They had an agreement that if one of them died, the others would buy his interest in the company. As John Freeman related in an interview years later, "Anderson knew that the enormous growth of the company could, one day in the future, result in its possible dissolution. The value of each interest had increased so much that any two surviving partners would have to almost dismantle the company and liquidate its capital in order to pay the taxes and honor the agreement between partners. Mr. Anderson made a decision he felt was best for the company, best for its employees—and certainly to the benefit of mankind in general."

In 1936, Anderson, whose health was beginning to fail, established the M. D. Anderson Foundation, which would be the beneficiary of his holdings in the firm. This would eliminate the need to break up the company because Anderson's stocks would pass to the foundation tax-free. He named himself and two attorneys, John H. Freeman and Col. William B. Bates, trustees. Freeman and Bates were partners in the law firm of Fulbright, Crooker, Freeman & Bates, which handled Anderson, Clayton & Company's legal affairs. Over the years, Bates and Freeman had become good friends with Monroe Anderson and the three had spent many hours fishing together.[6]

While Anderson was busy organizing his foundation, Dr. Elliott continued his efforts to build support for the Texas Dental College. After a speaking engagement in Pittsburgh, Pennsylvania, in 1938, Elliott stopped to visit the University of Pittsburgh campus. There he saw a newly completed, forty-two-story building, the Cathedral of Learning. He was so inspired by this building, which housed most of the university departments in one structure, that he returned to Houston and began to promote a similar structure to house a medical education and hospital complex. This is one of the first, if not the first, recorded public efforts to establish a medical center in Houston.

Elliott recalled during an interview years later, "In 1938, while I was at the dental school, I had come back to the University of Pittsburgh and saw this tower building. Well, I thought it would make a great idea for this [medical] tower business—so we developed a building. I had a student from Rice, an architectural student, who was over there getting his teeth fixed, so I took out the book I had and showed him a picture. I told him I had an idea like this for a dental school set-up with a medical school." The impoverished student happily agreed to do some design work in return for receiving his dental care. When the student returned with his drawing, an elated Elliott could not believe his eyes. "We named it the Memorial Center for Health Education," said Elliott. "The medical school, the dental school, the pharmacy school, and nursing school were on the bottom wing, which went up about six floors, and on top of that we had the hospital. We put the hospital up there to get it out of the humidity . . . it was [the student's] idea. That was about 1938, and we knew nothing about Col. Bates and Mr. Freeman and the Anderson Foundation. [The Anderson Foundation] had been set up in 1936, and Anderson was still alive until 1939." Elliott had a model constructed, and the dental students made miniature versions that were used to publicize his idea. For the next three years, Fred Elliott's crusade to establish a university affiliation for the dental college went hand-in-hand with his campaign for a comprehensive medical education institution in the city.[7]

A third part in the story of founding the Texas Medical Center was unfolding within the University of Texas. The school had launched a search for a new university president and also for a new dean to head the medical college (UTMB), which was located in Galveston. During the next six years, a fierce struggle for control of the University of Texas, its board of regents, and its Galveston Medical Branch at times threatened to overwhelm the fledgling Texas Medical Center. In his autobiography, Fred Elliott alludes to the political turmoil surrounding the brief tenure of Dr. John W. Spies as dean of UTMB in Galveston.

During the summer of 1938, the University of Texas carried on a search for a new president under the leadership of acting president Dr. John Calhoun. Simultaneously, the medical committee of the university's board of regents conducted its own effort to find a new dean for the University of Texas Medical Branch in Galveston to replace Dr. W. S. Carter, who was scheduled to retire on September 1. The three members of the board of regents medical committee included J. R. Parten, a Houston oilman; Dr. Kenneth Aynesworth, a surgeon from Waco; and Dr. Edward Randall, president of the board and also a professor at UTMB. Randall, age 78, was the oldest member of the board of regents. He had married into the family of William Pitt Ballinger, one of Galveston's most powerful and prominent citizens, and was well connected politically in the Island City. Randall had been on the faculty of the Medical Branch from its inception and had served also as the president of Galveston's John Sealy Hospital. He was described as "irascible, arrogant, domineering" in his later years, and it was said that he "acted as though he were solely responsible for the Medical School." During his long tenure at UTMB, Randall had become one of the most powerful citizens in Galveston, and he virtually ran the city's hospital–medical school complex.[8]

As a physician, Kenneth Aynesworth cared deeply about the Medical Branch and had developed serious concerns about the school's administrative organization and quality of education. The retirement of Dean Carter provided an opportunity to hire a new dean from outside the school who could implement the kind of reforms that would bring the administration back under the authority of the university president and the board of regents. The way the system had evolved over the years left the university president and regents with very little control over the Medical Branch or John Sealy Hospital. A committee of five faculty members elected by the faculty themselves managed the medical school, leaving the dean with little actual authority. The situation was much the same with the hospital. A five-member board of managers administered John Sealy Hospital, which was established by the estate of John Sealy in 1887 as a teaching hospital for the University of Texas Medical Branch. University regents appointed two board members, the Galveston city council appointed two, and these four board members chose the fifth person. In 1922, Sealy's son and daughter, John Sealy II and Jennie Sealy Smith, established the Sealy and Smith Foundation to ensure continued financial support for the hospital. Soon the trustees of the Sealy and Smith Foundation dominated the hospital's administration, relegating the University of Texas to an even lesser role in the hospital and medical school complex.[9]

In addition to his role as chairman of the board of regents, Dr. Randall held positions as a director of the Sealy and Smith Foundation and as a member of the hospital board. As historian Don E. Carleton has observed, "This convoluted administrative set-up and its overlapping and competing lines of authority had allowed Randall and a faculty clique to control the Medical School for years." Aynesworth's plan to hire a new dean from outside the medical school would work to give more authority to the dean and the university president. Conversely, a new dean also would reduce the autonomy that Randall and his cohorts on the faculty executive committee and on the hospital board had enjoyed for such a long time.[10]

The search for a new dean took its own peculiar twists and turns. The regents first turned to Dr. Tom D. Spies, a native Texan, who had made his reputation as a nutritionist at the University of Alabama School of Medicine in Birmingham. But Spies was reluctant to give up his research to become an administrator. He suggested that his brother, Dr. John W. Spies, would be a better candidate. John Spies had earned his bachelor's degree at the University of Texas and a medical degree at the Harvard University School of Medicine. Spies had an impressive record that included two years of study in Belgium and faculty appointments at the Yale School of Medicine and at the Peking Union Medical College in China, where he administered a Rockefeller Foundation cancer treatment program (1931–35). He also had administrative experience as director of the Tata Memorial Hospital in Bombay, India (1935–38). He held memberships in many scientific societies, including the Royal College of Surgeons and the American Association for Cancer Research.[11]

In August, 1938, Randall contacted Spies in India and arranged for him to visit Galveston for an interview with the regents' medical committee in October. But then Randall went to New York without Parten and Aynesworth to interview Spies himself. He invited Spies to Galveston and at a luncheon on October 28, 1938, Randall introduced Spies as "the next dean of the medical school." The faculty, who believed this was an introductory luncheon and not a "coronation," were shocked. Spies's appointment officially began November 1, 1938, but he was granted a leave until January 1, 1939, to wrap up his affairs and ship his belongings to Galveston. On December 28, 1938, the board of regents also named Dr. Homer Rainey as the new president of the University of Texas.[12]

The appointment of a new dean at the medical school was a hopeful sign to Elliott. As he recalled years later, "As soon as they appointed Spies, I immediately went to Galveston to start connections with him. Being new, I wanted to get to him before anybody else did. Right off we clicked because he had helped to establish a medical foundation, a medical school in Peking. And he immediately took on the idea of our dental school [affiliating with the University of Texas Medical Branch] since he had done the same thing in Peking."

Spies appointed Elliott to be a special lecturer in stomatology (dentistry). "I went down there once a week to lecture and he and I would get together and would talk about what he really wanted. Even way back then he said 'this

town is too small for a medical school.' He said the [medical] school ought
to be up at Houston. There was quite a little bit of personal conversation between the two of us." With new leadership in place, it seemed that the University of Texas and its medical school would enter the new decade with experienced, stable hands on the helm. But instead, a conflict was about to
erupt that would embroil both the new president and the new dean in a ti-
tanic struggle for control of the university.[13]

Edward Randall had hired John Spies to be "his man," hoping to have
control over the nature and extent of any reforms that might be implemented at the medical school. However, Spies believed that he had been
given a mandate from the new president, Homer Rainey, and from the
board of regents, as represented by J. R. Parten and Kenneth Aynesworth, to
reform the medical school and bring it under university control. This immediately put him at odds with most of the faculty, including Edward Randall and with Dr. L. R. Wilson, superintendent of John Sealy Hospital. Evidence suggests that Spies interpreted his mandate as a blank check to utilize
any tactics to accomplish his mission. The sense of power seems to have been
intoxicating and perhaps clouded Spies's judgment.

According to UTMB's *Seventy-five Year History,* "The day that he moved
into the dean's office, Dr. Spies ordered that the wires of the main switch-
board be tapped. A tape recorder was installed in his office in such a way that
it could be activated surreptitiously, and a hidden microphone was discovered and displayed publicly during the later famous 'Un-American Activities Trial.'" An ugly campaign began that lasted for about three years. During this time, John Spies was accused of everything including that he was
"immoral, dictatorial, professionally incompetent, verbally abusive, responsible for the suicides of two faculty members, a sex pervert, a thief, an anti-
Semitic Fascist, a communist, a Nazi sympathizer, a homosexual" and that
he had been forced to leave his position in India because of "his lecherous
behavior with the wives of his professional associates."[14]

On August 6, 1939, as the hullabaloo continued to grow at the Medical
Branch in Galveston, Monroe D. Anderson died. Although he had established the M. D. Anderson Foundation three years earlier, Anderson had
not provided specific instructions for the trustees on how the funds should
be distributed. Thomas D. Anderson, the nephew of M. D. Anderson, related that when his uncle died in 1939, "the bulk of his estate was poured over
into the hands of the trustees of the M. D. Anderson Foundation. And as
soon as the estate tax clearances and all were given, then the trustees had
about $20 million and they didn't know what to do with it." One of the

Anderson Foundation trustees, John H. Freeman, recalled that, "Mr. Anderson had some rather definite ideas as to its purpose, but nothing regarding specific activities had been put on paper. He came by the office almost every morning to talk things over. So Colonel Bates and I knew a great deal about what he had in mind, but his foundation gave pretty wide latitude to its Trustees, with the expectation that we would have further direction from him as we went along. He became ill and died before we could work out specific ideas with him, so we simply had general directions."[15]

During the fall of 1939 and into 1940, Anderson's estate was in the process of being probated. While these proceedings went forward in Houston, Dr. John W. Spies was fighting for survival as dean of the University of Texas Medical Branch on Galveston Island. By October, 1939, accusations by the medical school faculty brought down a full investigation by the board of regents on the doings of Dr. Spies. But after three days of private hearings, Spies was absolved of all charges. The university's president, Homer Rainey, assumed responsibility for the medical college, and Spies would now report directly to him instead of to Edward Randall, the university regent who also had represented the school. Rainey took a hard-line position with the medical faculty, and Randall threatened to resign from the board of regents. Ironically, Randall had essentially "railroaded" the hiring of John Spies, in the belief that he could control the new dean. But Randall was now engaged in a death struggle with his protégé for control of the Medical Branch.

In January, 1940, word spread about a proposal to create a cancer clinic for the Medical Branch under the supervision of Dr. Spies. Another idea also circulated that a new superintendent would be appointed at John Sealy Hospital and the board of managers eliminated. This move would bring the hospital under the control of the medical school dean. A furious Dr. Edward Randall submitted his resignation from the board of regents in protest, saying that he "could not subscribe to the radical reorganization plans . . . the abolition of the elected executive committee . . . a succession of radical changes in which departments were combined and reorganized without consultation or knowledge of the heads of the departments."[16]

The infighting continued unabated, and after yet another regental investigation in July, 1941, the board of regents announced its intention to fire John Spies from his deanship. Two weeks later the regents backtracked and renewed Spies's contract for two years. By November, the faculty had sent out a seventeen-page letter to alumni that concluded with an entreaty to contact members of the state legislature, University of Texas regents, and influential colleagues to garner support for the faculty's "Statement of Policy and Resolutions." Although President Homer Rainey opposed the faculty's proposals to change the governance of the Medical Branch, the board of regents conceded to the faculty and granted its approval in December, 1941. Still, the problems did not end.

In May, 1942, the Association of American Medical Colleges issued a twenty-five-page report and placed the Medical Branch on probation. The American Medical Association followed suit, observing that "the situation at the Medical Branch of the University of Texas is . . . a bitter and open fight between a majority of the medical school faculty and the medical school and university administration." On June 5, 1942, the board of regents fired Dr. Spies. Within four years, the same fate would befall Homer Rainey. Dr. Chauncey D. Leake replaced John Spies and in 1946, Dr. Theophilus S. Painter took over after Rainey's dismissal.[17]

During the formative years of the Texas Medical Center, from 1941 to about 1946, a great struggle for control of the University of Texas and its Medical Branch in Galveston raged like a fierce, unrelenting storm. In the midst of all this turmoil, Elliott deftly steered a course through the tangle of University of Texas politics. The significance of this in relation to the Texas Medical Center is that the Texas legislature would place the founding institutions, the M. D. Anderson Hospital for Cancer Research of the University of Texas and the University of Texas Dental Branch (formerly the Texas Dental College), under the purview of the University of Texas board of regents. Early plans called for the Houston institutions to be managed by the Galveston Medical Branch. Therefore, the struggle for control in the University of Texas system was such that the outcome of the conflict could have a direct impact on the scope and size of the Texas Medical Center.[18]

Generally speaking, there were five major steps, or building blocks, that led to the establishment of the Texas Medical Center during the early 1940s. First, in 1941, the Texas legislature appropriated $500,000 for the University of Texas to establish a cancer research hospital. Following this, the trustees of the M. D. Anderson Foundation seized the initiative by proposing to match the state's grant and to provide a suitable plot of land if the hospital was located in Houston.

A third building block appeared in 1943 when the legislature agreed to accept the Texas Dental College into the University of Texas system. Thus, the University of Texas M. D. Anderson Cancer Hospital and the University of Texas Dental Branch became the first two institutions of what was soon known as the Texas Medical Center. Also in 1943, the Baylor University College of Medicine (now Baylor College of Medicine) relocated to Houston and would become the first medical school in the Texas Medical Center. Later in the year, voters approved the sale of 134 acres of land adjacent to the Hermann Hospital for $100,000 to the M. D. Anderson Foundation. In 1946, the Anderson Foundation presented the deed to this land to officials of the Texas Medical Center, Inc.[19]

The most significant developments in the creation of the Texas Medical Center were the 1941 founding of what eventually became the M. D. Anderson Cancer Center, and the decision of the board of regents in 1942 to locate that institution in Houston. The cancer hospital became the first institution of what would develop into the Medical Center.

In 1941, when the Texas legislature first created the state's cancer hospital, the public perception of the disease was one of "an unmentionable and hopeless disease, to be whispered about in private but never discussed in polite circles." But physicians had begun to take a new interest in cancer during the early 1900s when they observed increasing life spans, which in turn meant that many people were living long enough to develop the disease.[20]

The death rate from cancer continued to increase, and in 1940 the Texas Medical Association's Committee on Cancer determined that the state needed to provide treatment for indigent cancer patients. The committee members met with officials from the state Department of Health and developed a new plan based upon legislation originally passed in 1929 that authorized the creation of a cancer hospital to be located in Dallas. Since the legislature did not provide any funds, the cancer hospital was never established. The Committee on Cancer referred their proposal to the Texas Medical Association's executive council to be considered for presentation at the annual meeting in May, 1941.[21]

At about the same time, one of the members of the Texas House of Representatives, Arthur Cato, a druggist from Weatherford, was about to introduce his own proposal to establish a state cancer research hospital. Cato's father and both of his wife's parents had succumbed to cancer. This personal tragedy inspired Arthur Cato to introduce House Bill 268 on February 5, 1941, to establish a state cancer hospital. The medical association's cancer committee quickly set up a meeting with Representative Cato to join forces and combine the two proposals into one bill. They also believed that the best course of action was to link the proposed cancer center with the existing cancer program of the University of Texas.

Arthur Cato needed the help of someone with medical expertise to write up the parts of his bill that related to medicine. Dr. John Spies, who was still dean of the University of Texas Medical Branch, had traveled to Austin to

lobby for an increase in the state appropriation for his budget. He learned of
Cato's desire to propose a bill establishing a cancer hospital, and the two men
got together to collaborate. John Spies worked with Cato on his original bill
and then with the Texas Medical Association committee to rewrite the bill
so that the new cancer hospital would be a part of the University of Texas
and the Medical Branch in Galveston. As Fred Elliott described the story
thirty years later, he recalled that, "Spies, being a bachelor, went to Austin
and set up a room with a closet full of liquor to push over the budget for the
medical school. He was asking for a sizeable budget to change over from the
$450,000 a year that Randall had been asking for so many years." Spies met
with Cato and told him about his previous experience setting up a cancer
program at the Tata Memorial Hospital in Bombay, India. "He told Cato he
would help him with his cancer hospital—if he would help him get his
money for Galveston," said Elliott. "So they made that deal."[22]

On May 29, 1941, the House of Representatives passed House Bill 268 by
a vote of 85-39, appropriating $1.75 million for the establishment of the
Texas State Cancer Hospital and the Division of Cancer Research. The senate reduced the appropriation to $500,000 and on June 30, 1941, Governor
W. Lee O'Daniel signed the measure. The legislation assigned responsibility
for the oversight of the cancer program to the University of Texas and its
board of regents. There was some opposition to the bill to create a state cancer research hospital. Many Texans believed that the United States soon
would be involved in World War II and thought that spending scarce dollars on non-military medical research was unnecessary and frivolous.[23]

John H. Freeman, a trustee of the Anderson Foundation, noted that they
had been searching for a way to utilize the funds that Monroe D. Anderson
left to his foundation. "We had nothing specific in mind at the start," said
Freeman. "We had cast about to see where and in what manner we might
best put this resource to work. Two or three things developed that led us to
consider health as a matter that needed attention. We were looking at that
idea when the Texas Legislature authorized a cancer research hospital for the
state in 1941." The announcement that the state had appropriated $500,000
to establish a cancer research hospital, and also had provided that additional
funds could be sought from other sources, was an inspiration to the trustees.
"That took our attention immediately," said Freeman. "We moved over to
that idea and away from what we had been thinking. We got in touch with
Dr. Spies and, through him, Dr. Rainey, the President of the University of
Texas in Austin."[24]

Anderson Foundation trustees, Dr. Rainey, Dr. Spies, and members of

the board of regents held a series of meetings to discuss the proposal to locate the new cancer hospital in Houston. John Freeman recalled, "Several of
them took place on the back porch of Colonel Bates' home on Brentwood
Drive. There was a ceiling fan there to assist the prevailing breeze—not
much air conditioning then, you know—and it was just a comfortable situation for relaxed conversation. Colonel Bates, Mr. Wilkins and I had met
there frequently after hours to discuss the affairs of the Anderson Foundation, and so it was just natural to invite these men to join us there from time
to time." The trustees agreed to provide $500,000 to match the funds pro-
vided by the legislature if the University of Texas would establish the cancer
research hospital in Houston and name it the M. D. Anderson Hospital.
The foundation also agreed to provide temporary quarters and twenty acres
of ground at an appropriate place in Houston on which to build a permanent hospital. The University of Texas board of regents accepted the proposal on August 8, 1942.[25]

The idea of establishing a medical center began to take a firm shape in the
minds of the Anderson Foundation trustees. "We then made up our minds
that we would try to put a [medical] center in here," said Freeman. "We
didn't envision anything like it is now, of course, but we wanted to put in a
sizeable center. We talked to the University of Texas about putting in what
would amount to a branch of the University's Medical School at Galveston.
We felt that with Houston as close to Galveston as it is, there could be a part
of that Galveston school in Houston."[26]

The birth of the University of Texas cancer hospital cleared the way for
Dr. Elliott to push for passage of a bill that would bring the Texas Dental
College into the University of Texas. In 1943, the state legislature authorized
the acquisition of the dental school by the University of Texas. During the
eleven years since Dr. Elliott had become dean of the Texas Dental College,
he had brought the school back from the brink of financial disaster and failure. On September 1, 1943, when officials completed the transfer and the
school became the University of Texas School of Dentistry, the dental college was free of debt and had assets valued at $150,000.

Together with the M. D. Anderson Hospital, the dental school formed
the nucleus of the medical center. "We were encouraged by the work of
Dr. Fred Elliott and others to bring Texas Dental College, located here in
Houston, into the University of Texas system," said John Freeman. "That
turned out to be an important factor in the creation of the medical center."
Dr. Ernst W. Bertner paid tribute to Dr. Frederick C. Elliott's work on behalf of the University of Texas Dental Branch during a speech at the UT

School of Dentistry several years later. "In addition to my warm personal regard for him, I want to declare that if credit for the development of the splendid University Dental Branch were to be measured by individual contribution to it, the major share of that credit should go without question to Dr. Frederick C. Elliott. The untiring efforts of Dr. Elliott have made possible the present honored position of this school, and his vision has had more to do with the planned future of this great institution than can ever be measured." The creation of a state cancer hospital in Houston and the assimilation of the dental college by the University of Texas meant that Elliott's dream to create a Memorial Center for Health Education was about to be fulfilled in a way that even he could not imagine. Instead of a single building reaching up into the sky, the idea immediately began to evolve into a much broader concept that ultimately became the Texas Medical Center.[27]

During the summer of 1943, the M. D. Anderson Foundation continued its efforts to establish a medical center in Houston. The Baylor University College of Medicine in Dallas had fallen upon hard times and trustees began to consider closing the school or relocating. When word of this reached Houston, the M. D. Anderson Foundation stepped up with a promise of $1 million for construction of a facility and an annual gift of one hundred thousand dollars a year for the next ten years if Baylor University College of Medicine relocated from Dallas to Houston. The medical school moved to Houston during the summer of 1943 and set up temporary quarters in a building formerly occupied by Sears & Roebuck until construction of a new facility could begin after the war.

The Anderson Foundation also purchased some 134 acres of land adjoining Hermann Hospital from the city of Houston. The plan was to develop the land for the Medical Center. The city acquired the acreage from Will C. Hogg, son of former Texas governor James S. Hogg and one of Houston's leading citizens. Hogg originally had purchased the land during the 1920s and offered it to the University of Texas Medical Branch at Galveston if the school would move to Houston. The Hurricane of 1900 devastated the Island City, and many businesses had since relocated to Houston to get away from the vulnerable Texas Gulf Coast. Some Houston business leaders thought it was time for the Medical Branch to move inland, too. But a host of legal restrictions and the city's powerful business and political interests would never permit the school to leave Galveston. Will Hogg then sold the property to the City of Houston at cost. Since the land had been intended as part of the city's Hermann Park, when the Anderson Foundation approached the city with a purchase offer in 1943, a referendum had to be called for the voters to approve the sale. Voters approved the referendum in December, 1943, and the Anderson Foundation took possession at that time. The foundation planned to provide plots of free land and some initial funds for building construction to institutions moving into the Medical Center.

After World War II ended in 1945, a number of hospitals began planning to relocate or build new facilities in the Medical Center. And when the Texas Medical Center was formally incorporated later in the year, the first signature on the charter was that of Frederick C. Elliott. Other signatories included James Anderson (not related to the family of M. D. Anderson), Hines H. Baker, William B. Bates, E. W. Bertner, Ray L. Dudley, John H. Freeman, Bishop Clinton S. Quin, and Horace Wilkins as incorporators. On February 28, 1946, officials formally dedicated the Texas Medical Center. The M. D. Anderson Foundation donated the 134 acres of land, and W. Leland Anderson presented the deed to Dr. Ernst W. Bertner, who had been named director of the Medical Center.[28]

The five men who formed the nucleus of what became the driving force behind the establishment of the Texas Medical Center—Anderson Foundation trustees Colonel William B. Bates, John H. Freeman, and Horace M. Wilkins, along with Drs. Ernst W. Bertner and Frederick C. Elliott—all had personal relationships and were all well acquainted with each other. Dr. Bertner lived on the top floor of the Rice Hotel and was a neighbor of John Freeman, who resided just down the hall. Wilkins was president of the State National Bank of Houston and had succeeded M. D. Anderson as a trustee of the Anderson Foundation in 1940. Freeman and Bates were trustees of the M. D. Anderson Foundation and also were partners in the same law firm. Elliott became a close friend of Bertner, and he knew Bates, Freeman, and Wilkins very well.[29]

In a moment of marvelous historical coincidence, a unique group of men found each other at precisely the right time and in the right place to fulfill their destiny of bringing a medical center to Houston. This cadre of Texas Medical Center pioneers had complimentary talents and shared a common interest to improve public health in Houston. In time, this interest manifested itself in a dream to establish a "city of health" like no other in the history of the world.

Frederick C. Elliott played a pivotal role in this magnificent endeavor. Stoic, disciplined, scholarly, and self-effacing—perhaps this explains, in part, the mysterious silence that has enveloped his career. In the eyes of some, he was only a dentist, not a medical doctor. He was not a gregarious fellow, in the mold of his friends Ernst W. Bertner, Ralph Cooley, or R. Lee

Clark. Yet he was an innovative teacher, deeply concerned about the state of public health in his adopted home of Houston, and also a man who loved to cook, travel, and write poetry. Dr. Mavis P. Kelsey, Sr., the founder of Houston's Kelsey-Seybold Clinic, knew Fred Elliott very well. "I guess you could call Fred Elliott kind of a Renaissance man," said Kelsey. "Although he was a dentist, he thought in terms of the entire health care profession. Dr. Elliott had a broader vision for Houston's health care."

Fred Elliott loved teaching and earned a reputation as an innovative professor of dentistry. World-renowned heart surgeon and medical pioneer Dr. Denton A. Cooley also knew Fred Elliott very well. Cooley, as a young man, entertained aspirations of following in his father's footsteps to become a dentist and recalled accompanying his father, Dr. Ralph Cooley, to dental conventions. Ralph Cooley had studied at the Texas Dental College and frequently lectured at the school. His acquaintance with Fred Elliott dated back to Elliott's arrival in 1932. "Through the years, Dr. Elliott was very close to my family and visited our home," Denton Cooley recalled. "We lived on Montrose and West Alabama, and Dr. Elliott frequently came by to visit my father. I think Dr. Elliott's photograph hung in my father's office there. So I have always had great respect for Dr. Elliott, and my mother loved him very much. She thought he was just a wonderful person."[30]

Ultimately, Frederick C. Elliott was a modest man with an extraordinary destiny. When he died on December 31, 1986, at age ninety-three, he was still involved in the health profession. More than eighty years earlier, he began his career in public health by helping in his father's drugstore. During his long lifetime, he overcame his share of obstacles, personal setbacks, and tragedy to fulfill his destiny as one of the founders and leaders of the Texas Medical Center. The chapters that follow are his recollections and observations of the early years of the Texas Medical Center. Dr. Elliott's service to humanity, his efforts to find ways to improve public health services and ease human suffering, and his quiet diplomacy in the midst of ego-driven, quarrelsome institutional politics are a fine example for his successors and an inspiration to all who share his deep love for the Texas Medical Center.

The Long Road to Houston

THIS IS AN AUTOBIOGRAPHY. I shall relate it in story form. Some of the dates, which I shall relate as I tell the story, will be approximately correct. Some of my assumptions will be probabilities. I believe that most autobiographies, biographies, and even some histories are, in reality, stories, so facts are not always facts and events are sometimes a wee bit colored. In this story I will, to the best of my knowledge, tell it like it was.

My father, Thomas Amos Elliott, was born in Whitney, near Loftus, Yorkshire, a small town on the east coast of England where my grandfather, James Elliott, was a tenant farmer and a Methodist lay-minister. He was a stern, self-disciplined individual who exercised discipline with all who came in contact with him. My grandmother, Sarah, my father and his two sisters, Annie and Ruth, always said, "yes sir" and "no sir" when speaking to my grandfather. My father worked in the small field and took care of the sheep and cattle. One of his two sisters, Annie, was a gifted natural musician who once entertained William Ewart Gladstone (prime minister of England) at the piano after Sunday services when the family later lived in the village of Quitby.

My father was still a lad when my grandparents immigrated to the United States, settling in Pittsburg, Kansas. As in England, landlords owned much of the land and "tenanted" it to immigrants who were but a cut above the peasants in the old country. By the time my father reached adolescence, my grandfather had saved enough money to buy a fifty-acre farm in Buhler, Kansas, which eventually he converted into a grape vineyard and apple orchard. My father and grandfather prospered on the farm, producing apple cider and vinegar. The farm produce was transported the four miles from Buhler to Pittsburg by wagon and team.

I do not have any record of my mother's place of birth, but I believe it was somewhere in Pennsylvania, about 1865. After her mother's death, her father moved to Pittsburg, Kansas, where her brother, Isaac Jenness, owned a harness shop. The mining industry purchased his harnesses since Pittsburg and the surrounding area was one of the chief sources of coal at that time. The mines used small animals of the donkey family they called mine mules. He also sold harnesses for the larger animals used on the local farm. My mother's father invested heavily in real estate, becoming a successful businessman. As a girl, my mother, Katherine Jenness, attended the public schools in Pittsburg. She entered Kansas Normal College in Fort Scott, Kansas, about 1883, and graduated in 1886.

My Grandfather Jenness frowned upon my father. He thought my mother, being a well-educated young woman more suited to city life, was too refined for my father. As a gentleman of means, he simply would not permit his daughter to be a farmer's wife. My grandfather doted on my mother, a petite, very pretty girl, and often called her "Kitten" and "Puss." My mother, however, was very much in love with Thomas Elliott and could not be swayed in her intent to marry him. As a condition to his consent to the marriage, Grandfather Jenness insisted that my father take up another line of work. However, my Grandfather Elliott was enraged at the prospect of losing a good farm hand and became estranged from his son. My Grandfather Jenness then set my father up in a combination bookstore-stationery shop in Pittsburg. When it appeared that my father was established as a merchant, he permitted my parents to marry in 1887. Alas! My father was not a good businessman even then. He pressed too fast, overextended himself, and became insolvent. My Grandfather Jenness had to step in and bail him out. About this time, mother's older brother, who was educated as a homeopathic doctor at the University of Pennsylvania, moved to Pittsburg, Kansas, to be near the rest of the family. As a solution to the improvident financial situation of his sister and her new husband, he convinced my father to study pharmacy. Once my father had obtained a state license to practice, my uncle and Grandfather Jenness set him up in a drugstore. Thomas Amos Elliott and Katherine Jenness's first child, Chesley, was born in 1888 and died of diphtheria in infancy. My brother, Francis, was born in 1890. I was born in 1893, and given the middle name of Chesley after their firstborn.

Though frail and often ill, my mother was a gentle woman, a warm and loving presence in our early lives. My father, like his father, James, was a stern disciplinarian, usually unable to show affection to Francis or to me. We lived in a small cottage my Grandfather Jenness built on the backside of his property. My grandfather lived at the front of this land holding in a large, impressive house surrounded by beautiful old trees and a fine fence. Occasionally, we would go to visit my father's parents in Buhler where we played in the orchards.

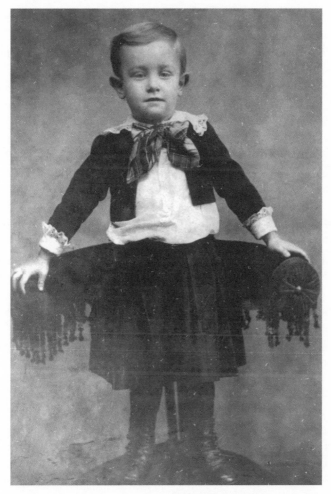

Earliest known photograph of Frederick Chesley Elliott at age three, standing on a chair.

Now, in my ninetieth year, incidents often stand out vividly in my mind's eye from my early childhood. A picture of my sweet mother's face, the smell of apples as I romped in the orchard, the sounds of the cider mill and press. When I was about four-and-a-half years old, I was put in kindergarten because my mother, before term in a fourth pregnancy, had taken seriously ill. My father found a hired girl to come in to town from the farm country everyday to do the housework and to take care of my mother. One day, while I was at kindergarten class, I looked up to see the hired girl rushing into the room and talking to the teacher. She grabbed my hand and dragged me along faster than I could walk to find my brother in another part of the school. The girl said that our mother was calling for us. We were frightened and rushed home as fast as we could. She died before we got there. Instead of her sweet voice, we heard the racking sobs of our father. It was a terrible time, which marked the true end of my babyhood and perhaps the beginning of my development into a serious, solitary child, always too eager to please.

After mother died, instead of returning home to play after school, Francis and I went straight to my father's drugstore to work. We cleaned up, carried trash, and mopped the floor. In the morning before breakfast, we built up the fire in the stove. At night, we did our homework near father as he filled prescriptions, banking the coals in the stove as our last chore of a long day. First Francis, and then myself, as we grew older, expanded our duties by rolling pills, filling capsules, and making deliveries. Each of us could accurately make up and fill simple prescriptions by our twelfth birthday. This introduced us to the Latin names of drugs and the apothecary measurement system. One of our jobs was removing old labels from used prescription bottles. After washing, these bottles were filled with father's "Bed Bug Killer," made from corrosive subliminate dissolved in turpentine. Householders periodically painted the poison around rooms and into creases in the furniture, cracks on the floors, and mattress ticking. On one occasion, I picked up an old, unlabeled bottle half-filled with liquid, which was too large to fill with bed bug poison. It was our habit to throw such discard against the brick wall extending beyond the drugstore. The purpose of breaking the bottles was so that shattered glass could accumulate and be carted away more easily. When I heisted the bottle by the neck to throw it, the contents ran down my arm, onto my shoulder. The bottle contained carbolic acid and I suffered a second-degree burn.

While it may seem by today's standard that Francis and I had a hard life under the watchful and demanding eye of our father, our life was pretty much the norm for midwestern lads at the turn of the century. Most of our school mates—whether farmers or townies as ourselves—worked before and after school. The rigidity of the times and the iron wills of our fathers were deeply imbedded in all our lives.

Stern though he was, my father possessed a sometimes less-than-subtle sense of humor. He would take an accountant's type of stool out in front of the drugstore when business was slack and just sit, chatting with passersby, taking a break from the drug work. Sometimes, when a customer left the

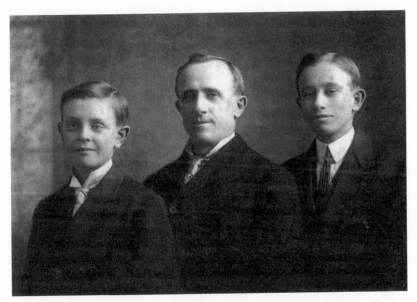

Young Elliott with father, Thomas Elliott, and brother, Francis "Frank" Elliott.

store, he would go back out and find some other person sitting on his favorite stool. This became rather vexing to him, so he conceived the idea of pouring carbon disulfide in the "hollow" of a substitute stool. If someone sat on the stool, their body warmth would warm the disulfide, generating a hot gas. After the interloper moved on, Father would switch stools and appear to be comfortably enthroned on the hot seat when the person passed back by. My father was also less pious than he desired Francis and me to believe. I recall that when the sex symbol of the day, Eva Tanguey, played Pittsburg, a "drummer" for the National Biscuit Company named Charlie Peoples invited her to my father's pharmacy for a "medicinal" dose of hard liquor.

If there was a place of emptiness in our hearts, it was that once filled by our mother. When our father remarried some years after mother died, Francis and I could never seem to forget that our father's wife was our stepmother. We let pass no fault or human frailty in the poor woman. Money was scarce, times were hard, and we associated our misfortune with her presence. This was in stark contrast to the bittersweet memories we had of a better life with our dear mother. Beyond the usual sibling rivalry there grew and flourished a compulsion in each of us to excel in our achievements in competition with the other, in the fruitless battle to win our father's approval. For me, it seemed always that my father favored Francis, the elder son. On the other hand, Francis remained convinced throughout his life that I was father's golden-haired boy.

Our father's drugstore stocked only patent medicines, prescription drugs, and accessories, with toiletries for the women and chewing tobacco and cigars for the men. While cigarettes were outlawed in Kansas, open saloons and houses of ill repute were common. It became my responsibility to make regular delivery of "specifics" to what I initially imagined to be an exclusive women's boarding house. My, but I thought those were the loveliest of creatures, so warm and nice, always caressing my cheek and brushing hair from my eyes with their long, slender, jeweled fingers. As I approached puberty, father forbade me to speak to the women in the street and he took over the deliveries.

The pattern of our days changed drastically again when I was about fourteen years old. Francis was an intelligent, studious young man. That year, at the age of seventeen, he passed the Kansas State Board of Pharmacy examination. While my father was so proud of Francis for that fine accomplishment, I felt he was somewhat put out with me because I was confined to a long period of bed rest. I was believed to have polio.

About that time, the coal mines around Pittsburg closed down after the miners went on strike, and the unions demanded that credit be extended to the miners. Many of them ran up large bills in the drugstore and then skipped out to greener pastures. My father could not weather the long-range effects of the strike. He went bankrupt and decided to relocate, admitting he could not afford to support Francis and me any longer. We were stranded in Pittsburg.

I went to Muskogee, Oklahoma, where I got a job in a drugstore. I led the druggist to believe I was eighteen years old. I was able to hold a man's job because of my experience in my father's store. In time, my father settled in Arlington, a small community in west Kansas where the local banker was saddled with a bankrupt drugstore. He allowed my father to take over the store on a monthly payout with nothing down. My father wrote to me asking that I come help him out in running the store. This Elliott drugstore had a soda fountain, which along with a front register, was my primary responsibility. In a town of four hundred people with but one doctor there was little enough profit from a drugstore to support my father and his wife, much less me.

Soon after I moved back with my father, I began studying for the state boards in pharmacy. In those days, although some larger cities had schools of pharmacy, independent study followed by examination still prevailed in rural areas. I studied after work each night. During my bout of polio, I had completed a school term successfully through bedside study, and I was confident I could succeed again at home study. In the fall of 1910, while still sixteen, I took the pharmacy exam and failed it by a good measure. My ego was grievously injured and my confidence shattered. In the wake of losing face before my father and people in the community who were aware of my effort, I swallowed my pride, gritted my teeth, and returned to my books. The following July, I took the pharmacy examination again, passing one-half point behind the first fellow. Sixty was the passing grade—I got 66.4. Of the fifty who took the test, twelve passed. Years later my brother showed me the letter my father wrote to him commending my tenacity and strong will with obvious filial pride and affection that I had never known he felt for me.

Though justified, because the drugstore could not support the both of us, I callously told my father I was too ambitious to be satisfied as his soda jerk and was leaving to earn a living as a licensed pharmacist. I soon found a job as a druggist in Greensburg, Kansas. After about six months, the owner of the store said he was expanding, opening another drugstore in Haviland, and he wanted me to manage it. The new store was in the west Kansas wheat country. It was situated in a small, unpainted frame building with a storefront porch. I built shelves down the center of the room that I loaded with the accessories brought from the other store. The first opportunity I had to demonstrate my capability as an independent businessman showed, instead, my enthusiasm and faulty planning in the form of collapsed shelving and shattered, broken merchandise!

After a while I got along alright. There was an excellent wheat crop that year and business was good. The only other drugstore in town was operated by a Quaker who refused to sell tobacco. Since I was not a Quaker, I had no qualms about it. Consequently, I got the summer farm and transient harvest business from the hands for whom chewing tobacco was a necessity. While they were about it, they picked up goods and sundries for the wife and kids. I started doing so well I put in a soda fountain. The next thing I knew the owner asked if I wanted to buy him out of the Haviland store on a monthly payment basis. At risk was the stock on hand, the future stock which I was to get from him, and the permanent fixtures along the walls that he had ordered from the showcase works. By this time, I had three part-time employees and a swelled head. Soon I wrote to my father and brother, telling them about *my* Elliott's Drugstore!

The next move was my triumphant return to Pittsburg, in the guise of a successful man of means, to win the hand of my childhood sweetheart, Anna

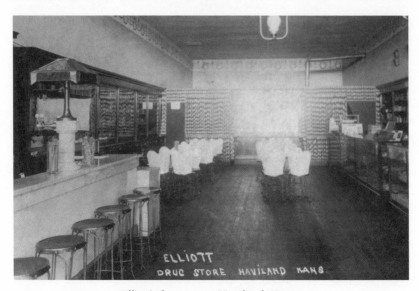

Elliott's drugstore in Haviland, Kansas.

Bracket. She worked as office manager for the Wholesale Candy Company and was, by the standards of the time, an independent woman. But, wooed and won, we married in 1914 and set up housekeeping in rooms behind my drugstore in Haviland.

That summer the crops failed. No rain, no wheat, no money, and no cash customers at Elliott's Drugstore. I had no choice but to extend credit to the folks who had been my making. Time passed and things did not get better. One morning I came to open the front door and met up with two men from the United States Court of Bankruptcy. They had been sitting on the stoop since daybreak just waiting for me to wake up and start stirring around. The very fellow who owned the store previously and had set me up in it in the first place forced me into bankruptcy. He was holding most of my paper, though there were other creditors. Since I was still a minor, my brother, Francis, was trustee for the small legacy left for the two of us by our mother. These creditors had nosed around in my past and dug up this asset, the only thing of financial consequence I had. Before the money could be attached, I had to go before the bench to have rights of majority conferred on me. My wife and I had to pack our few personal possessions and leave town. It was a sad and humiliating time.

In Glasco, a small town near Beloit in northwest Kansas, I gained employment managing another drugstore. The town dentist came in so often that we became friends. As we became familiar with each other, he took to ribbing me, asking why would I want to work so hard, just to make money for someone else? He would go on about only working nine-to-five with Sundays at home, making two hundred dollars a month, in contrast to my seven o'clock in the morning to eleven o'clock every night of the year on seventy-five dollars a month. Well, after a time, he got to me, or maybe it was his three hundred dollar Model A Ford. The only transportation I ever had of my own had either four feet or two wheels. So, you can see that dedication to a life of service to mankind was not exactly what motivated me finally to write to Kansas City Dental College. And part of it was that I did not want for my Anna to go on doing without and for me to have to go on grubbing for a living the rest of my life. Once notified that the school had accepted me, Anna and I worked and scrimped the rest of the year, pinching every penny, holding back all of the real money we could spare. All that spring and summer we canned fruit and vegetables in the half-gallon jars I brought home from the soda fountain.

When we arrived in Kansas City we had just seventy-five dollars over the amount needed for my tuition. We found a basement apartment in a tenement district near the school and paid two months rent in advance. I remember the dollar amount came to twenty-four dollars. Books and instruments cost sixteen dollars. Anna started looking for day work, and I looked for a night job. Then, just when our money cache had become so low that I was seriously considering quitting dental school, Anna found work. After I found a night job, I took to tutoring other dental students for pay and also became a teacher's assistant in the lab between my day classes for six dollars a month. Later, we found an attic apartment that was only nine dollars a month. We went from damp and dirty to high and hot. Since my wife worked on Saturday, I did our washing in the morning using a scrub board and galvanized tub in our landlady's cellar. In the afternoon, I would make up enough apple and ground meat pies to carry us through the following week.

By our third and last year, we could not afford to pay the dental school tuition. I had to ask my father-in-law to loan us the $150 we needed. Though Anna was still working and we were taking in two student boarders, we just couldn't make ends meet. After we had sold all of our furniture, piece by piece, we had to move in with my cousin. We were having a hard time, but we had a lot of reasons to be thankful. During the war in Europe, I had enjoyed a teacher's deferment with my only assigned military duty being at the student unit of the Emergency Medical Reserve Corps (EMRC) supervising study from six until nine each night. So many teachers had been pulled from school that I was teaching pathology, histology, and bacteriology because they could not get anyone else. In June, 1918, I graduated from the dental school with a 98.7, the highest three-year grade average ever achieved at that time.

My career in dental education began the day after I graduated from dental college. On that morning, I hurried to the college to pack my instruments, dismantle my "foot engine," and make other necessary arrangements to leave the school. I had just completed packing my clinic instrument case when Miss Ruth, as all the students affectionately called the dean's secretary, came to see me with a rather stern look on her face. She told me that the dean, Dr. Charles Channing Allen, wanted to see me. I went along with her, and she ushered me into Uncle Charley's private office. All students called the dean Uncle Charley because of their great admiration and respect for him, and also because of his charming personality. I did not know what was coming. He looked at me for a moment, then smiled and told me that he was pleased with my accomplishments while in college. He asked if I would be interested in a full-time teaching position in the dental infirmary. My salary, $150 a month, would be double the amount I had received when I last served as manager of a drugstore in 1914. I was agreeably surprised. In fact, for a moment, I was speechless. Then my short answer, "Yes. Thank you very much." It seemed that we had timed everything just right. I had accepted a faculty position at the school for the fall term, launched my career in dental education, and we learned that we were going to be parents in January.

The influenza pandemic, which played such havoc among the troops in Europe, came home with our wounded. It spread throughout the country, and everywhere people were sick and dying. My wife received a phone call from her folks in Pittsburg. Her sister was very ill. Her brother was very ill, too. Her family was having a tough time and telling her about it, so she came to me and cried and said she wanted to go home. My cousin warned me against letting her go. "You make her stay here," she said. Well, you look at me now. Can you see me making anyone do anything, especially in that kind of situation? Her family was close-knit, and I could refuse nothing Anna pled for. So she went.[1]

Anna was in Pittsburg tending to her folks when armistice was declared November 11, 1918. I recall this so well because Kansas City went crazy. People were running and screaming in the streets, shooting off fireworks and firearms. I had set up an old barber chair with a foot aid for a makeshift dental office in the front room of my cousin's house. Here, I used the chair to perform a little moonlighting dentistry for the neighborhood. I was sitting in the same place, resting after a long day of teaching and a few filling jobs at my chair, when I glanced casually out of the window and looked up the street. I was surprised to see Anna about a block away, walking slowly toward me. Without a call to me or a word to anyone in her family, she had walked out of her home in Pittsburg, taken the train to Kansas City, then the street-car out to the end of the line, and was trying to make it the last few steps home to me.

I was running to meet her before the reasons for her unexpected arrival penetrated. I wasn't even close enough to catch her when she fell in a faint to the sidewalk. She was a sight bigger than I was, and pregnant besides, so I do not know how I managed to carry her the rest of the way home. I was so frightened that all I could think of was how I could save my Anna. Alas, others also needed saving. No doctor could be found to make a house call, and there were no hospital beds vacant in the city. Hours later, a bed became available in a small, old, church hospital way out on Main Street. Only through the influence of one of the senior faculty at the school were we able to be bumped to the top of the waiting list, but it was too late. Our prema-ture baby died of influenza within minutes of his birth. That night, Anna, too, died of influenza.[2]

My cousin and I took Anna and the baby home to Pittsburg to be buried. I suffered a nervous breakdown. Dr. Allen and the rest of the faculty of the dental school rallied around me, providing encouragement and support throughout this period of devastating grief. In time, I resumed my full teach-ing schedule, throwing myself even more deeply into guiding my students in their academic and clinical pursuits. I became known as something of a firm taskmaster, pushing the boys further than they wanted to go. I was fre-quently ill and still bereft by the tragedy, which had overwhelmed me. My days were filled with students from dawn until late evening, when I dragged myself back to a cold supper at the boarding house near the school where I was now living. I had, by this time, attained the rank of full professor dur-ing my five years of faculty service.

In 1923, I decided that private practice was the thing for me. Although I remained with the college as professor of pathology and continued teach-ing on a part-time basis, I opened an office in the Wirthin Building in Kan-sas City. While there, I became acquainted with a gentleman on the second floor of the building. Although it was not more than a speaking acquain-tance, it was one that came back to my mind each time I saw one of his pro-ductions on screen and on television in later years. I am talking about Walt Disney.

After a couple of years, I again became dissatisfied and sold my practice to a young dental school graduate who had been in my dental pathology class. Although I continued to teach in the dental school, I did not return to the clinic full time. Instead, I joined the H. D. Justi Tooth Manufacturing Company of Philadelphia. My job was to travel to different cities, calling on dentists to explain the advantages of the Justi product over other products. The work was in the line of a pharmaceutical detail man, rather than a salesman. I was with H. D. Justi long enough to complete the educational campaign for the company.

Thereafter, I returned to private practice and established an office in downtown Kansas City. However, many dentists called upon me to consult with them concerning diseases of the mouth. The majority of these dentists had graduated from the Kansas City Dental School and had studied general and oral pathology under me. Many of these dentists referred patients to me with mouth diseases that they did not wish to treat. Beginning a practice in a downtown city such as Kansas City at that period was not too easily done. After many months of waiting and hoping, however, I did begin to receive referral patients from patients I was treating or had treated at some time. Unlike most practices today, a general practitioner then performed most of his own lab work. I did all of the lab work in the field of dentures, crown and bridge, and in-lay. I also baked my own porcelain jacket crowns. Compared to today, my fees were ludicrous. I performed many root canal operations for ten and twelve dollars, whereas today [1976], the same operation would be around $150 to $200.

In early 1928, I met Ann Orr, the sister of one of my patients. A petite, fun-loving flapper from St. Joseph, Missouri, she was considerably younger than I was, and I became enchanted with her immediately. She was so alien to the serious, professional-minded image I had of myself that I was just enamored with everything about her. We were married in the spring of 1928.[3]

After about three years, I had become dissatisfied with the private practice of dentistry. It was not possible to maintain both a high standard of excellence and earn a living. A great deal of time was consumed in the very delicate, tedious hand work of preparing various items that just did not pay off at the level I could charge for them. Also, I was offended by the lack of esteem awarded dental practitioners by both the public and the medical profession. I decided that private practice was not for me after all. Desiring a teaching career instead, I asked Dean Allen of the dental school to be on the lookout for a teaching or administrative position in another location. The college of dentistry at the University of Tennessee in Memphis sought recommendations for a good teacher from Allen. On his referral, I was offered, and I accepted, the position of associate professor of crown and bridge prosthesis in August, 1928.

The University of Tennessee schools of medicine, dentistry, nursing, and pharmacy were all located on a single city campus. I had my own research laboratory in the dental school and enjoyed the scholarly exchange with the faculty from the other university schools, as well as my responsibilities to my students. I saw, too, an opportunity for professional advancement that might not have existed for me in Kansas City.

I became quite interested in the study of the crystalline structure of metals and the effect on them during the casting process used in dentistry. The purpose of these studies was to determine the temperatures of metal and mold in order to control the amount of shrinkage that occurred in the casing process. My wife worked in the lab with me. She had artistic ability such that she soon was capable of carving teeth in wax as well, or better, than I. She became most helpful to me in the preparation of my teaching materials and in preparing my lectures for the professionals in the field. Ann became quite well acquainted with many of the faculty members of the school. They all became friendly with her, and she enjoyed her Memphis friends very much.

With the assistance of a fine dentist, Dr. Burrell Griffing, Ann and I developed many new methods of treatment, which I presented to the profession in that particular area of the United States. Because of my research and findings, I was invited to read papers throughout the country. My pharmaceutical background even led the dean of medicine to put the university drug room under my responsibility. I was in charge of all the university's alcohol, receiving ten or twelve barrels at a time, at a cost of about forty dollars a barrel. This was during prohibition, and we had to record the distribution of alcohol, by measure of the drop, for internal revenue purposes.

I enjoyed my work very much until one day when the dean called me into his office and said that the president had requested him to reorganize the departments of the university. I was let down by his announcement that it would be necessary for me to work under the professor of prosthesis, Dr. McCaleb, because I had expected to work into a professorship. When I told him that, he appointed me professor, but in one of the subdivisions of dental prosthesis.

Unfortunately, a conflict arose between the dental school and local practicing dentists that caused me to reassess my situation. At the dental school in Memphis, several others and I taught without a license to practice dentistry in Tennessee. The local dentists took exception to this. They thought our dean was too progressive and were concerned that there would be too many dentists in Tennessee. I was one of the faculty who was singled out for not being licensed in the state. Although an arrangement to rectify the situation was offered to me, I had become disillusioned because any deal I made would reflect badly on the dean who had supported me. I again began to cast out for another position in a new location.

This, I found, was not hard to do. Surprisingly, my reputation was so well known that many schools offered me appointments when they learned of my desire to teach elsewhere. I had offers from Georgetown University, the Medical College of Virginia, New York University, and, later, an offer from the Texas Dental College in Houston. Ann and I drove to Richmond to visit the Medical College of Virginia. We selected that school first because Dr. Webb Gurley had been employed in the department of operative dentistry two years previous to that time. The Gurleys had been good friends of ours in Memphis before Dr. Gurley left the University of Tennessee and accepted a position at the Medical College of Virginia. Ann felt that she and Helen, Dr. Gurley's wife, would have the opportunity to form a relationship in Richmond. We liked the school and the dean, Dr. Harry Bear, very much. Since Richmond was near Washington, D.C., Dr. Gurley drove Ann and I to Georgetown University where I had the opportunity to view the appointment offered me there and to look at the dental school. It was an excellent school, but I preferred Richmond to Georgetown, not only because of our friendship with Dr. Gurley, but also because of the school's excellent dean, Dr. Bear.

Later, Dr. George Powers, a prominent Memphis dentist, telephoned and invited me to have lunch with him. I presumed that he wished to talk to me about his son—a student at the college. During our lunch, Dr. Powers opened the conversation not about his son, as I had expected, but about my decision to teach elsewhere. Dr. Powers told me that he was a member on the Council of Dental Education and president of the Tennessee State Board of Dental Examiners. He told me that he had visited the Texas Dental College in Houston to make a study of the school for the council. The school had been private and only recently, in 1929, was established as a public trust school. He said the school was in bad shape and that it needed a dean who could get it into a position where the council would recognize it. He said the council members did not believe the school should closed because it had a nice group of dentists on the faculty, private practitioners, and a nice new building. He also said that there was a need for a good dental school in that part of the country and then asked if I would be interested in the deanship. This was rather startling because I had not thought of becoming the dean of a school—I liked teaching. Naturally, I was flattered by his consideration. While the other offers were far more financially attractive, none of them offered a deanship, which appealed to my desire for professional recognition.

I thanked Dr. Powers and told him that I would be glad to visit Texas and discuss the appointment with the president of the college. I drove to Houston while Ann stopped in Fort Worth to visit her sister. After a night's rest at the Sam Houston Hotel, I drove down Fannin Street to the dental college. As I approached the dental college on that lovely July morning, I was pleasantly surprised to see a new building that seemed to have been built especially for the school. This was not the case in Memphis or in Kansas City. The buildings in those two cities were old and had been remodeled for use as dental colleges.

Aileen McNaughton, the appointment clerk, introduced me to Elna Birath. I spent considerable time with Mrs. Birath during my stay in Houston. During our conversations, I learned that she was the only administrative person at the dental college. She was in the dean's office, but her appointment was bookkeeping and accounting. I was impressed with her gracious manner and the quality of her conversations. Mrs. Birath suggested that she would like to show me the building. As we walked through the clinic, I noticed that the equipment was modern—much better than the equipment that I had used previously in Memphis or in Kansas City. Mrs. Birath introduced me to Dr. Percy Wynn and to Dr. Raymond Snider, both of whom were part-time teachers. She also introduced me to Dr. Robert Robinson who was the technical instructor for the freshman and sophomore students and the only full-time teacher in the college. These teachers were young, and, as I learned later, they were all excellent dentists.

In my conversation with Dr. Powers at our luncheon, he mentioned to me that the classes were small. However, when I learned that Dr. Robinson was teaching two classes, it puzzled me because I had been accustomed to teaching only one class of fifty or sixty students. When I mentioned this to Dr. Robinson, he smiled and explained to me that the total number of students in both of the classes that he was teaching was less than thirty students.

The next day I met with Dr. Finis Hight, president of the Texas Dental College Board of Trustees, Dr. Walter Scherer, and other members of the board, to discuss with them the appointment, which I was considering. I was told that my salary would be $300 a month, beginning October 1. This was much less than I had received in Memphis and much less than what was being offered to me at the other two schools I had visited. However, this did not disturb me since it was the challenge rather than the salary that interested me.

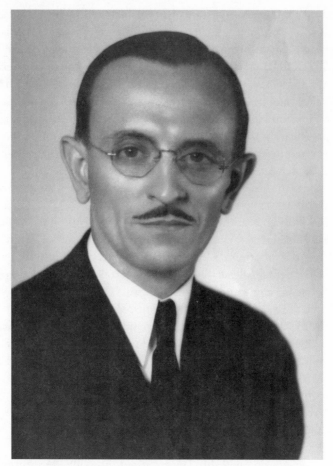

Elliott as dean of the Texas Dental College, circa 1932.

Later, after I had returned to the hotel, Dr. Hight called me and informed me that the members of the board unanimously wanted me to come be dean of their college. I told Dr. Hight that I would consider the appointment further, and that I would write to him after I had had the opportunity to discuss it with my wife. Also, I explained to him that I wanted to consider their offer as it compared to the other two offers I had received. As we drove back to Memphis, I discussed the Houston appointment with Ann. We decided that Houston offered us the best opportunity for growth, even at the lesser salary. I accepted the position as dean of the Texas Dental College, effective September 1, 1932. I was almost thirty-nine years old.

Texas Dentistry, Public Health, and the Texas Dental College

~

EARLY IN THE HISTORY of Texas as a state, there was a recognized need for better health education facilities. Attempts had been made to establish a private university with a medical college. In 1844, Hermann University was organized but never opened. Soule University was organized and began operation in Chapel Hill, Texas, until it closed in 1856. Prior to its closing, a committee was appointed by the university president to determine the best location for the medical school, which would be re-established. In a choice between Houston and Galveston, Galveston was chosen. Dr. Ashbel Smith of Houston was a member of the committee and, in 1850, had most likely played a prominent part in establishing a Houston institute to train young practitioners for the Gulf Coast area. Houstonians had raised twenty thousand dollars for the institute, demonstrating early on that they were generous in their support for medical projects. It was not until 1865, though, that the Galveston Medical College, a private school, began operations.

There was no state university in Texas yet, although several attempts had been made. No doubt, lack of funding was the principal reason for this failure, but there also was opposition to a state university. An attempt was made in 1857 to establish one, but the move failed. The failure may be attributed in part to a report that was presented to the House of Representatives by their education committee. A section stated: "Let those who may wish to receive what is called the genteel polish of a 'finished professional education' not call upon the people in the humble walks of life, upon whom they may in the future show their skill, fleecing or physicing, to pay for educating them. Let us not have doctors or lawyers manufactured by a state institution, and I say it in all becoming respect to gentlemen of the learned professions. God knows we have enough of them in the country, with a rising prospect for more of the same sort."

Despite opposition, in 1881, Texans approved a state university and a medical school. Heated debates became common throughout the state. There were citizens in every large city who clamored for the university to be located in their community. By the vote of the people, the main branch of the university was located in Austin, and the medical branch was located in Galveston. Houston was the principal contender for the medical branch, but not chosen by the voters. Galveston was the largest city in Texas at that time, and soon better instruction in clinical education would be available. The Galveston Medical College would close its doors, and in 1890 the Galveston Medical Branch was organized. Five years later, there was an attempt made to include a dental department as a part of the Medical Branch.

Sometime during the year of either 1838 or 1839, two physicians—Dr. Chapin and Dr. Harris—presented to the board of trustees of the Baltimore Medical College a plan to establish a department of stomatology (dentistry) in the medical college. Long before this move was made, Pierre Fauchard (1678–1761), had published *Le Chirurgien Dentiste ou Traiti des Dents,* in 1728. His book resulted in continued improvements in the methods of dental treatment, both in France and in the United States. Many dentists from the United States went to France to study the methods of Fauchard. It was probably Fauchard's teaching that resulted in the attempt by Chapin and Harris to establish a department of stomatology in the medical college. It was their feeling that stomatology should be included in the education of a physician, therefore, it should be taught in a medical school. They recommended to the board that a department of stomatology be established as soon as possible since the practice of many of the dental artisans was becoming a serious medical problem. Neither the board of trustees nor the faculty of the medical school approved the recommendations. They stated that they did not believe stomatology should be a part of a reputable medical college. Drs. Chapin and Harris were not to be frustrated by the officers and faculty of the medical college, though. They established a separate school for the education of dental surgeons. In 1840, the Baltimore College of Dental Surgery, the first college of dentistry in the United States, opened its doors.[1]

Dr. M. S. Merchant, who was to become a member of the faculty of the Texas Dental College, was an 1893 graduate of the Baltimore College of Dental Surgery. From Giddings, Texas, Dr. Merchant was one of the first members of the Texas State Board of Dental Examiners. He was appointed to this position by Governor Culberson on September 13, 1897, and reappointed by succeeding governors for each of the sessions until 1903. Sometime during the late months of 1905, Dr. Merchant resigned from the State Board of Dental Examiners to assist in the development of plans for the organization of the Texas Dental College.

Five years after the 1895 opening of the Medical Branch in Galveston, two bills were introduced in to the Texas state legislature. The first bill, Senate Bill 114, introduced on January 30, 1895, was an act to provide for the regulation of the practice of dentistry in Texas. The bill required applicants to be graduates of a reputable dental college or university. It failed to pass. The second bill, Senate Bill 217, was introduced on February 27, 1895. The title of this bill read, "An Act to Provide for the Support and Maintenance of a School of Dentistry of the Medical Department of the State University of Texas." It would provide fifteen thousand dollars for the support and maintenance of a school of dentistry for the years 1895 and 1896. Although the senate finance committee reported the bill favorably to the floor, it, too, failed to pass.

The failures of these two bills could possibly be charged to the pressure of a dental lobby, dentists who had not graduated from a reputable dental college and were fearful of college graduated dentists. Also, there may have been some opposition from a group of physicians who, like the physicians in Baltimore, did not believe that dental education should be a part of professional medical education.

At the next session of the legislature, House Bill 190 was introduced on January 18, 1897, to provide for the control of the practice of dentistry. It was similar to Bill 114 introduced in 1895, but it did not require the candidate to be a graduate of a reputable dental college. The bill came to the floor of the house on March 16, 1897. It passed both the house and the senate and became law on September 1, 1897. It was not until much later, in 1919, that a diploma from a reputable dental college was required to practice dentistry in Texas.

Once again, thirty-two years later, it appears that another attempt was made to establish a state operated dental college. On April 16, 1927, Dr. W. O. Talbot of Fort Worth, Texas, appeared before a committee of the Texas Legislature to testify regarding the advisability of establishing a dental department at the state university. There is no information as to whether a bill for the purpose as indicated was introduced in the house or the senate. Whatever was done, no dental department of the university was authorized at the 1927 session of the legislature. Interestingly, the resolution introduced by Dr. Talbot made no reference to the Medical Branch in Galveston. It was intended that the school be an independent branch of the university, such as the Medical Branch. I believe that this resolution read by Dr. Talbot must have been prompted by the board of trustees of the Texas Dental College, since it was followed closely by the introduction of another bill introduced by the trustees of the college just four years later. At the 1931 session of the legislature, a bill to create a dental college as a separate branch of the University of Texas was introduced, and was closely related to my appointment as dean of the Texas Dental College in 1932. But first, I will relate the birth of the Texas Dental College.

Early in 1904, at a banquet in Beaumont, Texas, John Henry Kirby mentioned that Texas should have a dental college for the education of the young people of Texas, since at that time there was not one in state. Kirby was one of Houston's most enthusiastic, civic-minded citizens. He was active in many other civic enterprises and in state affairs that were helpful to the people of Texas. Some of the prominent dentists of Houston, after learning of Kirby's address, began discussions with him concerning a dental college for the city. They discussed their plans later with many prominent physicians in Houston, one of whom was the president of the Harris County Medical Society.[2]

From this group of physicians, laymen, and dentists, the first board of trustees of the dental college was selected. While Dr. Merchant, who had become one of the prominent dentists of Texas, was among the group to discuss the possibility of a dental school for Houston, he did not become a member of the board, since at the time he was still a member of the State Board of Dental Examiners. In the fall of 1904, the board of directors was appointed. At their first meeting the board authorized the appointment of Edward S. Phelps to draft a charter of incorporation for the Texas Dental College. Later, on February 11, 1905, a meeting of the board of directors was held in Dr. Olympio F. Gambati's office. At this meeting, the charter was approved and the secretary of the board was instructed to mail the charter to the secretary of state, requesting him to certify the Texas Dental College as a state of Texas corporation. A few days later, a charter of incorporation was received, then two hundred certificates of stock were printed, each for fifty dollars a share, and a seal of the corporation was obtained. The Texas Dental College was formally on its way.[3]

Just seven days later, at the same meeting place, the by-laws were adopted and a faculty—all of whom were physicians, dentists, and other scientists of Houston—was appointed. It appears that Dr. Walter H. Scherer was not one of those who developed the plans for the dental college, nor was he elected as a professor. However, Dr. Scherer later became a professor and a member of the board of directors, which he chaired on two different occasions. His name appears frequently in matters concerning the dental college.[4]

Professors were to receive a salary of one hundred dollars per year and the demonstrator of anatomy was to receive fifty dollars a year. These salaries would be paid provided that funds were available. If not, the faculty members would be given a promissory note. Twenty-eight years later it was necessary that I ask all part-time faculty members to serve without salary. They did this gladly. When I reviewed the meetings of the board of directors, I was surprised to see that the secretary did not record any board member statements concerning the items under discussion, nor did he report the actions taken. Also, I was surprised at the frequency of the board meetings. The board of directors devoted many hours to these meetings, since there was much to be done to hasten the opening of the dental college. They had to procure a building, purchase equipment and supplies, and place advertisements in dental magazines and in daily papers so prospective students would know that a dental college was about to open in Texas.

On February 5, 1905, the board met and selected a committee to search for a building suitable for a dental college. An advertising committee also was appointed. Seven days later the board met and approved the recommendations of the advertising committee. At this meeting they authorized the secretary to send notices to the newspapers, to issue circular letters, and to advertise in the two Texas dental journals that were published at the time. He was given permission to purchase a safe, letterpress, and letter file. Also, the building committee reported that they had located a structure to house the dental college. The building owner prepared a lease for the second and third floors to be reviewed by the board. On March 25, 1905, the board of trustees approved the lease and authorized the building committee to make any alterations that were necessary for the operation of a dental college. The building was located on the corner of Congress and Travis, across the street from the farmer's market.

In this short space of time, only seventeen days since the first meeting of the board of trustees, a building had been located and leased, supplies and equipment had been purchased, and a faculty had been appointed. The building committee reported that at the meeting of the trustees on April 1, they had completed their plans for the alterations required. The committee was authorized to take bids and proceed with construction, provided the cost would not exceed five hundred dollars. The equipment ordered cost a thousand dollars.

On June 3, 1905, Dr. M. S. Merchant was appointed to the faculty of the college as a demonstrator in the infirmary (at this time all dental school clinics were called infirmaries). He would receive a salary of one hundred dollars a month, to work on a full-time basis (8 A.M. to 5 P.M.) each day until the college started its first school year. Then his teaching hours would be changed to half time. His appointment began on August 1, 1905. Dr. Williams and Dr. Gambati completed the copies of the school catalog in the latter part of June. It was approved by the trustees and ordered to be printed. Those who had worked so arduously for the epochal day, the first day of school, were becoming excited as it approached.

The first faculty meeting was held on September 5, and classes started on October 2, 1905. Several students who desired to transfer from other schools had been accepted in the upper classes. It was these same students who served the first patient who came to the college infirmary for treatment.

During the spring of 1906, it seemed that too few patients were coming to the dental college. Patients were needed for the students' education. Also, without a sufficient number of patients, clinic revenue would not be sufficient to cover the operations expenses of the college. The school had to depend upon the clinic receipts and student tuition to operate. The board of trustees was concerned and instructed Dr. Merchant to prepare in writing ways and means by which more clinic patients might be secured. At a later meeting, the secretary was instructed to place an ad in the labor journal. He also was instructed to print cards that would entitle the holder to one "amalgam filling and cleaning free." At the end of the first school year of the college, R. T. Atlee became the first graduate from the college, receiving his Doctor of Dental Surgery degree.

How the Texas Dental College managed to survive is puzzling. Beginning with only one graduate in 1906, and then through the years to the beginning of World War I, the number of graduates each year averaged only fourteen students. But in the fall of 1918, the number of students entering the freshman class increased. The dental college moved to larger downtown quarters to accommodate the growing number of students. Seven years later, the college moved a second time. The board of trustees decided to construct a building for the dental college and chose a site at the corner of Blodgett and Fannin. The Alumni Building Company was formed and charged with the responsibility of financing and building the new building, which was completed in 1925. The new building, no doubt, helped continue the increase in the size of classes.

During the years prior to the completion of the new building, Dr. Walter H. Scherer had been serving as president of the board of trustees. While the status of the dental college as a recognized college had not been changed, the number of privately operated dental colleges in the United States began to decrease quite rapidly. Dentistry was beginning to be recognized as a pro-

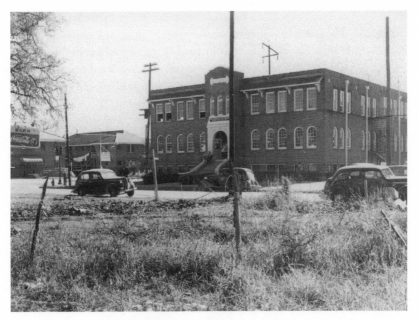

Texas Dental College, late 1940s.

fessional education that should be a university discipline. Harvard University, the University of Illinois, and many other major universities throughout the United States were including dental education in their curriculum.

The Texas Dental College's board of trustees, recognizing this trend, moved to have all the properties owned by the Alumni Building Association transferred to them, after which the college was to become a public trust institution. This transaction was completed on March 21, 1929. Just a few months later, on August 5, 1929, construction began for a second story and basement addition to the dental college building. All of the actions taken by the trustees between the years of 1925 and 1929 were directed toward improving the teaching facilities and strengthening the instructional program so that the requirements of the American Dental Association's Council on Dental Education might be met. Otherwise, the college would be forced to close.

In 1927, Dr. George Powers, a personal friend of Dr. Finis Hight's, visited Hight at his home. It was during his visit that Hight sought Powers's advice as to what other actions the trustees should take that might convince the legislature that the University of Texas should pass the dental college bill that had been introduced earlier in the year. Representative Duval, from Tarrant

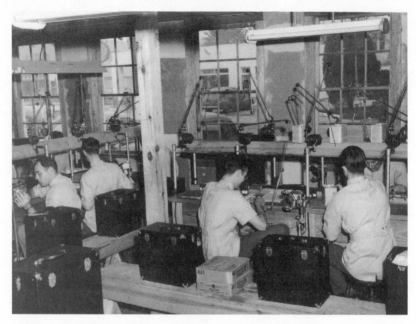

Technical Science Laboratory, Texas Dental College.

County (Fort Worth) had introduced a bill to this end. On April 16, 1927, Dr. W. O. Talbot of Fort Worth, who represented the board of trustees of the college, read a resolution to the House Committee on Education that explained in detail the advantages that the state would accrue if Duval's bill passed. It appears that the committee did not support the bill, which was unfortunate because the college's enrollment was higher at this time than it would be later. However, freshman enrollment was dropping even though the board had improved the educational facilities of the college. For the 1930–31 session, only ten students applied for admission to the freshman class. In the same year, twenty-four students would graduate, leaving only fifty-four students to start the next year in the upper classes. The lowered enrollment and the lessened revenue from the clinic resulted in a total income of only $20,334 for the year. The annual report made to the board of trustees that year was most discouraging, especially since it reported liabilities in excess of thirty-eight thousand dollars.

No doubt the failure to pass the Duval bill in 1927 aroused the interest of the Medical Branch in Galveston, renewing their desire to build their own dental school. An article that appeared in the *Galveston News* on December 6, 1930, reported that the Medical Branch would introduce a bill in January,

1931, for the construction of an addition to the Medical Branch's laboratory building for a state dental college.

At the Texas Dental Society meeting on May 23, 1930, a resolution from a committee was presented by Dr. Bush Jones, chairman, and approved. The resolution recommended that the Texas Dental Society support the plan submitted by the University of Texas Board of Regents! All members of the committee were prominent Texas dentists. Several local dental societies throughout the state endorsed the Galveston plan. At this meeting of the Texas Dental Society, the president appointed a new committee to confer with the board of regents of the university. This committee consisted of E. W. Smith of Dallas, J. F. Clark of Beaumont (one of the first graduates of Texas Dental College), W. B. McCarty of San Antonio, R. C. Cooley of Houston (a graduate from the Texas Dental College and a member of the Texas Dental College Board of Trustees for some time), Russell Markwell of Galveston, and T. A. Anderson of Corpus Christi. The committee presented the resolution of the Texas Dental Society to the board of regents.[5]

Fortunately, the officers and faculty of the dental school had not relaxed their efforts in this direction following the 1927 failure. Plans had been made

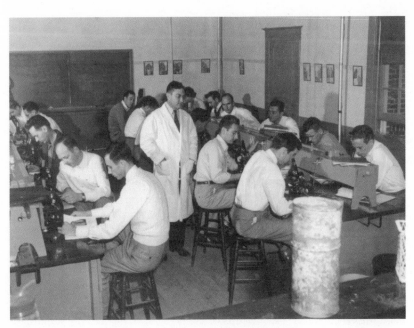

Science Laboratory, Texas Dental College.

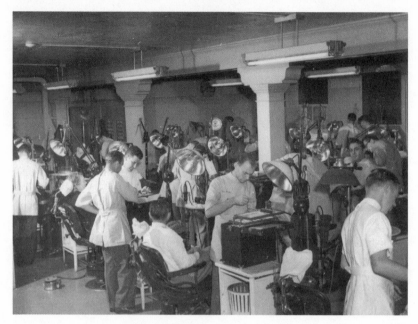

Dental Clinic, Texas Dental College.

to introduce another bill at the 1931 legislative session. Immediately after the announcement of the Medical Branch, an all-out drive for support of the Texas Dental College bill was started. Dr. Harry Cloud, executive dean of the college, strengthened his plan of action. Dr. Cloud was most effective and thorough in his direction of the effort, and his strategy was well planned. Yet he knew that it would be an uphill battle, for which the Medical Branch had set the stage. Dr. W. O. Talbot of Fort Worth reported to Dr. Cloud that he had learned from a member of the board of regents of the University of Texas that the board had met in Galveston in May, 1930, and discussed the plan for a dental school in Galveston. This meeting was not made public. During the discussion they had considered Houston as a possible location for the college, but by ballot vote Galveston was selected.

Dr. Cloud had not learned of this action until December 18, 1930. Some would have thought that this was the time to throw in the towel, but this was not so for Houston or the dental college. Houston was not then, and still is not, that kind of a city. *Houston Magazine,* a Chamber of Commerce publication, carried a story in January, 1931, concerning a visit by a prominent planning executive, R. H. Weisbrodt. In his remarks, he used the statement, "the amazing city of Houston." He marveled at the city's spirit of teamwork.

Already the Chamber of Commerce had offered to give all-out support for a University of Texas dental college in Houston. The president of the Chamber of Commerce appointed a committee of their members: Hugh Potter, Dr. Finis Hight, John Henry Kirby, Gen. Jacob Wolters, and Dr. F. A. Heitman. Dr. Heitman, a graduate of the Texas Dental College, never practiced but instead had entered the hardware business. This committee, and other prominent citizens of Houston, planned the legislative strategy.

On March 27, 1931, the committee appeared before the House Appropriations Committee in support of the Texas Dental College plan. A committee supporting the Galveston plan was also present. Colonel W. B. Bates, J. A. Phillips, Dr. Finis Hight, Hugh Potter, Dr. Harry Cloud, and Dr. W. H. Scherer represented the Chamber of Commerce committee. Members of the committee representing the Galveston Medical Branch plan were members of the board of regents from the University of Texas, members of the Galveston faculty, and citizens of Galveston. Colonel Bates, in his remarks, said that, "Houston paid the largest amount of state taxes, but had no state institution." Speaking for the Galveston committee, Dr. Edward Randall of Galveston, a member of the board of regents, said, "If the legislature gives us the $50,000 appropriation we are asking to establish this department of dentistry at Galveston, by 1932 the dental school of the university will open and by 1933 a new dental building of the most modern type will be on the university campus in Galveston." He continued, "The time is approaching when dentistry will necessarily be a part of the medical profession and if men are trained in the Galveston school, they will be well equipped to take their place among the scientific men of the world."

On May 15, 1931, the newspapers announced that the Texas Dental College bill was "killed" in committee. Likewise, the Medical Branch's request for an appropriation to build an addition to the laboratory building failed to pass out of committee. The House committee took this action even though the dental college and its supporters had exerted a tremendous effort.

On January 6, 1931, Dr. and Mrs. P. T. Breene, on a vacation trip, stopped off in Houston. Dr. Breene was a member of the Council on Dental Education. While in Houston, he received a wire from Albert Midgely, secretary of the council, stating that all members of the council agreed with him, therefore, the Texas Dental College had been granted a "provisional B rating" under certain restrictions. He asked Dr. Breene to notify the authorities of the Texas Dental College. The trustees deeply appreciated the action of the council, but it was not enough. It is evident that the strong opposition of the University of Texas Board of Regents to the Texas Dental College bill, in addition to support they had received from a large number of dentists throughout the state, resulted in the action that was taken by the House Appropriations Committee.

At the House Appropriations Committee hearing in March, 1931, Dr. Tom Coyle, president of the Texas State Dental Society, and Dr. Smith made the recommendation to locate the dental school in Galveston. At this meeting, E. M. Crone, a member of the board of regents, used the argument in support of the Galveston plan that "a vote of the people located a medical branch in Galveston and that dentistry is a branch of medicine." A wire story from Austin that appeared in the *Houston Post* on the morning of February 13, 1931, read in part, "The Texas Dental College is operated and controlled by Dr. Charles Edge. What his object is in tendering his valuable institution to the state for operation on the mere condition that the state pay off the $45,000 debt could not be ascertained here Thursday. The opinion was expressed that should the state locate the school in Galveston, it would put Dr. Edge out of business." Dr. Charles Edge was one of the group that formed the first board of trustees of the college. He had served as secretary and treasurer of the board from its beginning until 1931. He resigned from the board and the faculty of the dental school some time during that year. It could be that the heated meeting of the Texas Dental Society held in Houston in May, 1931, was part of the reason for his resignation.

This was the state of affairs that the board of trustees of the Texas Dental College faced at the close of 1931. The Texas Dental College still was not a part of a state university. It had an enrollment of only fifty-four students, a total income of approximately thirty thousand dollars for the year, and liabilities of over thirty-eight thousand dollars. This was the situation waiting for me when I assumed the deanship of the college in August, 1932.

Our household furnishings were packed for shipment by rail and had been put in storage until we located living quarters. The first order of business when we arrived in Houston was to find housing that would be within my income. To my surprise I learned that a dentist friend of mine from Kansas City, Dr. Walter Cronkite, Sr., was living in Houston. He left Kansas City about the same time that we moved to Memphis. Naturally, I was pleased to learn that someone I had known in Kansas City was living in Houston. He told me in a telephone conversation that he had read in the *Houston Chronicle* that I was coming to Houston. Later, we visited with the Cronkites in their apartment on West Alabama. In our conversation, I learned that he had just severed his connection with Dr. Finis Hight, president of the board of trustees of the dental college. Dr. Cronkite had made plans to return to his home in St. Joseph, Missouri, to practice dentistry. His son, Walter, Jr., had grown into quite a handsome young man. I had last seen him as a small boy. Later, for a short time, Walter, Jr., delivered the daily newspaper to us. He was just finishing high school, after which he attended the University of Texas in Austin. Walter, Sr., and his wife showed us around Houston and helped us find living quarters that were to Ann's liking and in keeping with our small income. But even though my salary was small, it made a large dent in the income of the dental college.[6]

As Ann and I became better acquainted with Houston, we grew to like it very much. We were tremendously impressed with the cleanliness of the city, especially the clean, smudge-free office buildings and the clean windows of the homes and buildings. We had been accustomed to living in coal burning cities. The friendliness of the people we met was refreshing. It seemed to us to be more like a small town. They did not have the rather distant attitude of the people in Kansas City, which was also noticeable to a degree in Memphis. However, in Memphis, this attitude changed to a friendly one when we lost some of our Yankee habits.

When I learned of the work that Mrs. Elna Birath had been doing, I came to the conclusion that she was a jack-of-all-trades. She was carrying out the administrative responsibilities of a dean, a business manager, and a building superintendent. She had only three other full-time employees to help her. She possessed an unusual ability to successfully carry out every project that she started. Dr. Joseph Arnold, brother-in-law of Dr. E. W. Bertner, served only as a part-time dean and could not devote the time necessary to the day-by-day activities. I now realize that if Mrs. Birath had not been as helpful as she was, had she not given me continuous encouragement, I might not have remained in Houston. Miss Winnie Fitzgerald was full-time custodian of the clinical dispensary. She, too, had multiple responsibilities—dispensing supplies as well as keeping watch over the operations of the dental infirmary.

The dental college had one office, which was for the dean. Mrs. Birath and I shared this office. This arrangement was a fortunate one for me, since it made it possible for me to discuss matters that were unfamiliar to me with her. I also could mention ideas to her whenever they came to my mind. She jotted them down and reminded me of them later. From our conversations I was beginning to recognize the serious financial condition the college was in. This was my immediate concern, a distressing one, since the income that the college received from the tuition of the very small student body and the revenue from the clinic did not meet the college obligations and the operating expenses.

I should have viewed the enrollment of only forty-eight students total in all the classes as an impossible situation. Yet, I did not. Since the beginning of the new college year was rapidly drawing near, our immediate task was to increase the number of students to be admitted, if this were possible. When I arrived only ten students had matriculated in the freshman class. I concentrated on one idea that I thought might be the best source of more students. I wrote a letter to all the students that I had taught in Kansas City and in Memphis and asked each of them to recommend prospective students to our college. This was a large order, since I dictated a personal letter to each student. Mrs. Birath had the onerous task of typing each letter. Time meant very little to us. An "eight hour day" was an expression that was not in our vocabulary, or, for that matter, in the vocabulary of our full-time personnel. They were just as concerned as Mrs. Birath and I were about our financial situation. I made it a point to keep the staff informed. After-hours, holidays, and weekends were a part of our work week. Discouragingly, the letters that I wrote to the graduates did not help. The replies that I received indicated that we were too late. Ten students were admitted to my first entering class.

Our days were spent discussing at length the financial situation that confronted us. Receipts for the year would not be sufficient to meet the outstanding obligations. How were the salaries to be paid, and how were the day-to-day operating expenses to be met? Such a condition called for a factual approach. We had to inform all creditors about our financial situation and seek their help. The bank, which was holding a large note, the dental supply houses, the mortgage holder, the paving company, the dental manufacturer who had furnished the clinic equipment in the new annex—all of them had to be informed. This was done, where possible, by personal visits. Otherwise, I wrote special delivery letters to them.

It was the depression years, and the times were on our side. The indebted properties would have been of little value to the creditors during this time. As a public trust institution, there were no individuals that were responsible for the liabilities of the college. The creditors agreed that their only hope for compensation was to follow the plan that we suggested. Mrs. Birath had developed cordial relationships with the principals involved before my arrival. These relationships had a great deal to do with the creditors believing that we could make it if they would allow us the time necessary to increase our enrollment. The creditors knew that this was the only source of revenue for us. Also, the confidence that our creditors had in the officers and faculty of the college was, I am sure, a major consideration when they accepted our plan. They, too, were a part of this unusual "teamwork city."

Some time later, I had the unpleasant task of asking each faculty member who lectured part-time to do so without pay. I explained to them the reasons why I had to make such an unusual request and they readily agreed. The salary that they would forgo was only one hundred dollars a year. It had become generally known that the college was in serious financial difficulty. There were doubts as to whether the college could even continue to operate. No one mentioned this to me, except one dentist who made the remark to me one day, "Why did you come to Houston? Had you not done so the college would have closed." I accepted this as an expression of his confidence in my ability. Much later, I pondered his real meaning. The arrangement that Mrs. Birath made with our creditors was a "pay-as-you-could" plan. This was done on a dogged month-to-month basis for several years. It was rather difficult at times, but happily, we were successful.

We devoted many hours to developing plans that might increase student enrollment in the college. It is possible that the many outside activities I engaged in helped our cause. My educational connections in Kansas City and Memphis were well known. My service as a member of one of the planning teams of the Curriculum Survey Committee was also well known. The recommendations were a topic for discussion by dental societies, state boards of dental examiners, and university faculties throughout the United States. The recommendations emphasized the importance of a university connection for all dental schools. The favorable reception that the report received also was a factor in improving the standing of our college. I was called upon more and more to lecture to dental societies throughout the United States. I made it a point to mention the names of prominent members of our faculty who at sometime earlier had lectured to the society before which I was appearing. This, too, served to strengthen the position of the college.

Our enrollment grew slowly. The additional income permitted us to increase our payments to our creditors. To rid the college of debt was almost an obsession with Mrs. Birath and me. Yet, we knew that this was not enough. The college must have a sound educational base. It must be a part of a university system, whether privately endowed or publicly operated. Rice Institute, as an endowed institution, seemed to me a logical choice. I discussed this idea with Mrs. Birath. It was essential that we have a university connection. This was a movement that was gaining momentum throughout the United States. It had become almost a demand of the Council on Dental Education that all dental schools should become a part of a university.

Now, for the first time, I learned from Mrs. Birath that an attempt had been made in 1931 to accomplish this purpose. The board of trustees of the

Texas Dental College had offered the school to the University of Texas. She explained to me in detail all of the events that had happened that she believed caused this attempt to fail. Immediately I thought this door was closed. I continued my discussion with her about the other possibility—Rice Institute. She pondered the idea for a moment and then expressed that it would be a difficult task—one that would require an extreme effort. Still, it was my conclusion that if a university connection was to be established, it was necessary to consider Rice Institute, since at the time it seemed to be the only hope we had. Mrs. Birath saw that I was troubled. I believe it was at this point in time that she asked me a surprising question. "Now that you know where we stand," she said, "I'd like to know the answer to a question that came to my mind when you first accepted this appointment. Why did you come to Houston?" I did not remember the question or my reply until many years later when Mrs. Birath related this incident to me and said that my reply to her was, "I had a dream." What I "dreamed," I cannot remember.

Many days followed during which I made inquiries of a few people in Houston and elsewhere about the Rice Institute connection. My inquiries brought the same response—it was worth a try. The next question: how to proceed? Mrs. Birath and I discussed many plans, but in the back of my mind I knew the Texas Dental College must improve its image if it were to be given a thought by a faculty such as the one of Rice Institute. Mrs. Birath agreed with me and expressed the opinion that this was a key factor in the failure of the University of Texas to accept the dental college in 1931. While we had made some progress in improving the image of the dental college as far as some departments were concerned, it was not enough. They were improvements known more by the members of the profession than by the public. It was necessary that Houstonians knew the Texas Dental College as a school that could be admired as much as Rice Institute. If the college were to become better known and appreciated by the people of Houston, then I, as dean of the college, must become associated with community agencies that were engaged in health and social welfare activities. Mrs. Birath paved the way for me. I was asked to serve as a member of the Council of Social Agencies in 1933. This membership led to appointments to boards and committees of other agencies that were members of the council.

These appointments came in rapid succession. First, in 1934, I was elected to the board of trustees of the Community Chest and later I served as chairman of the budget committee. I served on the board of the Houston Chapter of the American Red Cross and also on several committees. I chaired the Home Accident Committee, the Highway Safety Committee, and the Annual Roll Call. Later, I was appointed a member of a newly formed Houston Polio Committee. Ike McFarland served as chairman of the committee; Norman Beard of the Chamber of Commerce was secretary; and W. S. Patton, Dr. Joseph Poster, George Wilson, and I were the other members. This committee was organized during the beginning of the March of Dimes program at the time the polio epidemic was raging throughout the United States. It was severe in Houston. Our committee provided iron lungs for both Jefferson Davis Hospital and Methodist Hospital.

I also served as chairman of the Transient Relief Committee, which was a three-city committee for Dallas, San Antonio, and Houston. This committee took charge of developing ways and means for handling many of the transient, destitute people who were seeking employment in these cities. The depression was at its height, and it was irritating to members of our committee that other large cities in the United States were providing transients with tickets to Houston and other Texas cities, but no further. We did not appreciate their method of overburdening us with their problem. Later, I became a member of the board of the Houston Safety Association. George Wilson was chairman and Norman Beard served as secretary. The Houston Safety Association was interested primarily in industrial and highway accidents. As chairman of the Highway Safety Committee of the American Red Cross, I was interested in having these two committees work closely together.

I also served as a member of the board of the Houston Anti-Tuberculosis League, of which Dr. Elva Wright was chairman and Emmiline Renis was executive secretary. The dental school was able to offer the services of students for the cast of characters in a local radio broadcast, "The Doctor's Office," over radio station KXYZ, sponsored by the health committee of the Chamber of Commerce. These broadcasts were helpful during the Christmas Seal campaigns conducted by the league. All social agencies in Houston were vitally interested in the health activities of the city. They knew the condition of the health department and its woefully inadequate facilities. Therefore, it was necessary for them to provide services that should have been provided by the health department. At almost every meeting of the Council of Social Agencies, a member of one of the agencies would express the frustrations that confronted them whenever they asked the City Health Department for assistance. The services they needed were not available. Many times it became necessary for the Community Chest to establish new agencies to meet existing emergencies. One of the agencies created because of this reason was the Girls' Home School. Mrs. Quin, wife of Clinton S.

Quin, bishop of the Episcopal Diocese of Texas, was chairman of the board of this school, and I was one of the board members. I believe this school was operated in conjunction with the Houston Independent School District (HISD). The HISD physician served as the physician for the Girl's Home School which was established for one purpose: to provide care for children who had major venereal diseases. These children were between the ages of six and twelve. Older children were treated in the Health Department clinic. The educational needs of the children were provided by the school district. The hundreds of Houston citizens involved in the work of the Community Chest, the Council of Social Agencies, and other charitable health agencies in Houston were widely responsible for the health matters of the city. An aroused, community-wide interest in better health for Houston also was of immense value in promoting the welfare of the dental college. Interest in health matters by the people of Houston has never subsided.

Along with my committee duties, I was engaged in many other activities. I became a member of the Chamber of Commerce some time during 1933. This connection was to become a most important one because of the events that followed. I was invited to become a member of the Houston Rotary Club. Later, I was asked by the Texas State Dental Association to serve as chairman of a committee of which Dr. W. O. Talbot of Fort Worth and Dr. Monte Garrison of Wichita Falls were members. Our report to the Texas State Dental Association recommended changes that served later to improve dental services in all Texas state hospitals. The Texas State Dental Association had been requested to make this study by the State Hospital Board.

My services on the various boards of the social agencies and the board of the Community Chest served me well, educating me in the field of total health care. The needs that each agency provided to the less fortunate and to the general community seemed to me primarily a total health care need, a need which could be provided better by a total care health program. R. H. Fonville and his wife both served on many different boards of the Council of Social Agencies. I became well acquainted with them through these connections, as well as through the common interest that Fonville and I had, since both of us were druggists. Fonville operated the first prescription pharmacy in Houston, and the dental school purchased drugs and supplies from his pharmacy.

A little later, in 1937, Fonville became mayor of Houston. After the election, one of his first moves was to look at the structure and operation of the Health Department. What he found caused him to take immediate action. He asked the city attorney to draw up an ordinance creating a board of health as soon as possible. He learned the next day that an ordinance for a board of health already existed. Mayor Fonville telephoned me a little later and asked if I would serve as president of the board of health. I accepted. A few days later he called again and read a list of the members he wanted to appoint to the board and asked me for suggestions. I told the mayor that I hoped that all would accept and each of them did. The mayor appointed Dr. William Bertner, Dr. Judson Taylor, Dr. Henry Petersen, Dr. Philo Howard, Dr. Goldie Hamm, and Dr. Mylie Durham, Sr., all of whom were well-known and prominent Houston physicians, as members of the board. Ultimately, we were to become involved in a series of events, which we did not foresee, that were to make history for Houston.

I called an early meeting at the mayor's office. This was done so that we could learn firsthand what the mayor expected us to do. What we learned was that we would be performing our duties in the most trying circumstances. The summary of the mayor's findings as he related them to us caused us to realize that we were faced with critical conditions, if not dangerous ones. Fortunately for the board, the city council accepted our recommendations that a new city health officer be appointed. They appointed Dr. John Brown, both a physician and a public health officer, whom we had recommended. He made a careful study of the public health situation in Houston and presented a lengthy report to the board. It was not a pretty picture and needed immediate action. The board authorized Dr. Brown to prepare a request for the funds necessary to implement the most urgent needs. Dr. Brown and I presented this request in person. Although the request was presented to the council as an emergency, the council referred it to a committee. Later, the council voted down our request even though the mayor had made a strong plea with them to approve the recommendations.

It was obvious that drastic measures must to be taken, but our hands were tied. We could not make a move without the approval of the city council. Our board, we learned, was only advisory to the city council. Should we resign, or should we seek other ways to proceed? We did not resign. We sought a solution. Discussions with many prominent citizen groups in Houston led us to one conclusion: we would stay. We explained our dilemma through many public meetings. This gave us a little more suggestive power with the city council. They approved plans, which were brought to them by Dr. Brown, for the establishment of a detention clinic to be operated by the Health Department. The clinic would confine prostitutes until the volunteer physician working with Dr. Brown could release them, free from venereal disease. The clinic had wide public support. It would also serve those who could not afford a private physician.

An incident occurred, while not seeming too significant at the time, later started a chain of events that I believe played an important part in helping give birth to the Texas Medical Center. My position as president of the board of health was not a pleasant one. I was bombarded constantly by calls from irate citizens who needed public health services but were unable to get them. They made repeated requests to the Health Department for corrections of widespread unsanitary conditions that existed in Houston. One of the most common complaints was the presence of human excreta in drainage ditches.

One day, one of these irate citizens, Miss Georgianna Williams, came to my office at the dental college and demanded that something be done at once about our disgraceful, unsanitary, dilapidated treatment clinic for venereal disease patients. To her, a board of health that would operate a treatment clinic in an old, deteriorating, dirty building with nothing but tin washbasins where doctors washed their hands, old bed sheets hanging on iron pipes to separate the treatment rooms, tin pails with dirty water and paper towels in them, was a disgraceful situation. I listened quietly as she went on to say we should do something about all this or the board should be discharged.

Then, after her anger had subsided somewhat, she explained that she had taken her chauffeur to the clinic for treatment. She wanted to see if his description of the conditions that he related to her was true. It was and this was her reason for coming to me. I explained to her that though the appearance of the place was bad and the conditions that existed did not make it easy to maintain an aseptic condition, the doctors were quite meticulous in their use of these facilities. I also explained to her that the board could do nothing else. It was up to the citizens to do something about health facilities if they wanted better ones. She asked, "What can we do?" My reply to her was, "Better health facilities can be provided only through better government."

I did not know what a dynamic and determined person Miss Georgianna Williams was. She was responsible for rallying Houston women to fight for the necessary changes in city government. They adopted the slogan, "Better health through better government," and their drive was on. They circulated petitions and purchased billboard and newspaper advertising. They made house-to-house contacts and successfully circulated petitions to call an election. A new plan for city government was established—a city manager plan. An entirely different group of citizens were elected for mayor and city council—the same type of men as Mayor Fonville—sincere, honest, and hard working. The voters chose Otis Massey, a prominent businessman, to be the mayor of Houston. City council consisted of prominent bankers, businessmen, and lawyers. This group of citizens was in office only two years, how-

ever, it was long enough to start Houston toward a well-managed and efficient City Health Department and toward being a city better informed
about health.

During the period that I served on the board of health, I became chairman of a subcommittee of the City Charter Commission. The subcommittee recommended changes that were needed to improve health facilities.
Among our recommendations were a new city-county hospital and five
community health centers to be operated by the City Health Department.
Through much of this, what Mrs. Birath and I had started out to create, a
better image for the dental college, had been accomplished.

It seems that I was always, at the proper time, guided into fields of ex-
ploration that were to serve purposes unknown to me at the time. On one
of these occasions, the president of the American Dental Association asked
me to serve on a special committee to develop a plan for dentistry similar to
the Blue Cross/Blue Shield plan of operation. The board of trustees of the
American Dental Association approved the plan we developed. Each member of our committee was asked by the trustees to seek approval from his local dental society to implement the program in the committee member's
city. It was hoped that at least one city would start the plan so that other dental societies throughout the United States would establish similar programs.

The plan provided for an agreement with patients for dental services for
their children. It was not to be a group plan, such as the one developed by
Blue Cross. Each patient who accepted the agreement would pay a stipulated monthly charge, which could be paid by the quarter or by the year, and
would be made to a central office established by the local dental society. In
the beginning the plan would provide dental services, including orthodontic treatment, for children ages three to twelve. Since the dental society
would have no funds to begin the program, it would be necessary to gain
support from a foundation during the program's early years. When I returned to Houston, the idea seemed like such a good one to me that I immediately sought help from one of the foundations that was in existence in
Houston at the time. I did this before appearing in front of the Houston District Dental Society to present the plans for their approval. The officers of
the American Dental Association thought that if support for the program
could be provided before presenting the plan to the dental society, it would
be more readily accepted. I called the president of the Houston District
Dental Society and informed him of the plan that the American Dental Association was recommending. He suggested that it be put on the agenda of
one of the dental society's early regular meetings.

Following my report of the special committee of the American Dental Association to the members of the Houston Dental Society, I was astounded by the reaction of the members. To them it was a preposterous proposal. They criticized me severely for having presented such a report. I tried to explain to them that I was reporting for an American Dental Association committee. At the time, my explanation did not lessen their resentment towards me. I learned from the other members of the committee that they had received similar reactions from their local dental societies, but not quite as severe as the reaction I had received.

None of the dental societies accepted the plan. All but one member of the committee was criticized by their local societies as being in favor of "socialized medicine." Each of the members felt the same—never again would we serve on a committee where we devoted so much time for the profession, only to receive severe criticism. However, the appointment to this committee served as an education to me since I learned more about how group service plans operated. The director of the Blue Cross plan and health officials from companies that were providing services to their employees gave our committee complete detailed explanations on how their plans operated. The failure of this plan did not lessen the need for services to low-income individuals. I was compelled to continue to think of some type of plan for those needy people that might be acceptable to the profession. Houston needed to provide better health to these individuals.

A plan was developed that would provide services to those who were applying to many of the social service agencies, such as Jefferson Davis Hospital and other no-pay or low-pay clinics. It did not parallel the American Dental Association committee plan, therefore, to identify it, we called it "The Houston Plan." The plan would have established a city-operated agency that would provide professional services that were recommended and operated by the Harris County Medical Society and the Houston District Dental Society. The central clinic, with branches located throughout the city, would serve patients who applied for treatment. Patients coming to social agencies for health care would be directed to the central clinic. Needs would be studied and income levels established. They were to be classified as "no-pay," "one-fourth pay," "one-half pay," "three-quarter pay," or "full pay." The fees established were for low-income patients only. Preliminary clinical examinations would be made so that patients could be sent to the proper service agency or to a private practicing physician who would have agreed to provide services.

The patients understood that they would be required to pay the doctors' fees. They could, if it served their purpose better, apply for a monthly pay plan. The central clinic would manage these plans for the physician. Patients would be required to furnish proof that they were a low-income person or family. The plan was not accepted by the physicians and dentists of Houston, because it, too, was considered a method whereby socialized medicine might, as it was explained to me, "put its foot in the door."

We then developed another plan, which I read to the board of health at one of our meetings. The members of the board agreed that it was a good idea to try, since it was an idea that could help all people throughout the state of Texas. It was an educational plan with the purpose of informing the public, giving them facts about health matters, as well as explaining the "fads" that they should avoid. The membership of the Health League of Texas, as it was to be known, would be limited to physicians, dentists, public health officials, nurses, and druggists. The Health League of Texas was chartered but not implemented due to unavailable funds that would help acquaint professionals with the advantages of membership—the only means of support for the league.

The final chapter in my public health work was my appointment to the Texas State Board of Health in July, 1941, by Governor W. Lee O'Daniel. I became personally acquainted with the governor in a conversation with him on the night of his daughter's wedding reception. I was surprised to learn that my family had bought milk from his father when the governor was a very small boy in Arlington, Kansas, where my father operated a drugstore. I served on the State Board of Health until the dental school became a part of the University of Texas on September 1, 1943. It was then necessary that I resign from the board since I could not hold two state appointments.

During the time that I was associated with all the various health agencies in Houston, the dental college had provided emergency dental services to these agencies when they were needed. Likewise, the full-time employees, students, and many of the part-time faculty members were involved in the preparation of material for many of the programs that these agencies had underway. It was a real teamwork accomplishment in which I served only as the go-between. How to establish a sound educational base for the dental school continued to be the foremost question in our minds.

I became well acquainted with William Kirkland, chairman of the First National Bank, and a member of the city council. He was also a member of the Rice Institute Board of Trustees. I asked him one day what he thought about the possibility of giving the Texas Dental College to the Rice Institute for them to operate as their dental school. He told me that he would make informal inquiries. Later, he told me that although the Rice board members with whom he had talked were favorably impressed with the dental school, Rice Institute would not change their educational objectives, which were in fields foreign to health services. The dental college was getting along well, so our concern was not for operations as much as it was for what action the Council of Dental Education might take if the college did not become a part of a university.

Connections with the University of Texas and the Rice Institute appeared hopeless. The only door that remained slightly ajar was to seek support from a large private foundation. Perhaps the idea of developing an educational facility for all those who desired to enter the many health service fields would be more appealing to a large foundation than a dental college. Why not establish one common education center? This was an idea that warranted careful consideration.

Politics, Public Health, and the Origins of the Texas Medical Center

DURING THE 1930S, the dental college continued to make progress slowly. We were able to keep our heads above water. Also, I continued to make my national contacts by attending all meetings, which I felt was important to the college. I gave lectures throughout the United States at national and state dental meetings, as well as other associations that were related to many of my activities in public health and safety. At some meetings, I took side trips to visit colleges or individuals that I believed would be of help with projects that we had underway or were planning. I made a stop in the spring of 1938 at Pittsburgh, Pennsylvania. At the time I had only one item that I wished to discuss with the dean of the University of Pittsburgh College of Dentistry, but this stop proved later to be an important one. When I was leaving the dental school, I asked the dean about the beautiful building across the street. He said that it was the university. I asked him what college of the university needed such a large building. He smiled and told me that all of the colleges of the university except medicine and dentistry were in this one building. I expressed surprise, so he offered to show me through the building. It was an amazing plan. As I thought about this building on my trip back to Houston, an idea came to me. Why not house all educational disciplines related to health in one building?

Several days after my return to Houston from Pittsburgh, a student came to my office to ask about a patient. This patient was a graduate student in architecture at Rice Institute and was in need of extensive dental treatment. The college required payment in advance for their clinic services. Because of limited funds, the patient could not meet this requirement. Since the patient was a friend of the dental student, the student wanted to provide the service. He asked me if it were possible that this student be allowed the privilege of making monthly payments. A thought came into my mind, and I told him that there possibly was an arrangement that could be made where the patient would not be required to pay for the services he needed. The student was pleased, as well as surprised, and I asked him to bring the patient to my

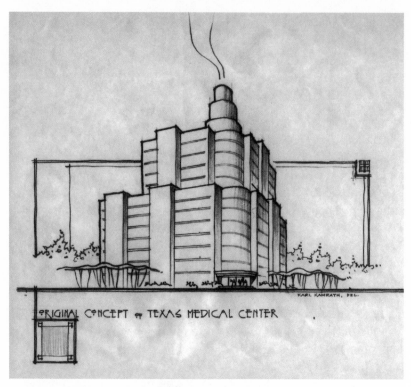

Architect's drawing of Elliott's idea for a medical center, the Memorial Center for Health Education, circa 1938.

office. I described the building at the University of Pittsburgh to the patient. He knew of this building.

I explained to him that what I had in mind was a building for a "university for health education" only. I suggested that it should be of similar design as the building in Pittsburgh but that I wanted several changes that would make it a functional facility for the education of all health professionals. Several weeks elapsed, then one day the student brought to my office an architectural rendition of a beautiful tower building. A special faculty meeting was called at which I displayed the architect's rendition of the building. Then, I sprung the surprise. I informed them of the total plan for which the building would be used. Their reaction was a most favorable one. Likewise, when the architect's rendition was shown to the student body and its use explained to them, they too were pleased.

Dr. Bob Robinson suggested that a model should be made of this sketch which he believed would be more impressive than the colored rendition of the architect's, which had been sketched on a piece of corrugated cardboard cut from a shipping carton. Dr. Robinson's idea was excellent and he proceeded to develop the model. When completed, the model stood about three feet high. Most impressive was Dr. Robinson's reproduction of the "Torch of Eternal Health," which I had mentioned to him as a creative idea similar to the war memorial in Kansas City, Missouri. Dr. Robinson demonstrated the model to a small group of us, and, to our surprise, the "torch" operated. He had placed a pan of water over a Bunsen burner, which produced steam that was emitted from the top of the building's tower. It was lighted by a small flashlight, which he had placed inside of the building. It looked very much like the war memorial tower in Kansas City. We were delighted.

Mrs. Birath asked Dr. Robinson if it would be possible to make a small model similar to the large one. When he asked her how this model would be used, she said that she wanted all of us to use it when we gave talks to civic groups and at other meetings. We wondered why the larger building would not be best. She explained that a small mold should be made of the building, then the buildings poured from the mold could be used as place card holders at luncheons. This was a large order, but not too large for Dr. Robinson. He enlisted the aid of all the students in his classes to pour hundreds of models from several molds he had made.

In late 1938 and 1939, many Houstonians were talking about the Memorial Center for Health Education. While this was a medical center, as physicians, dentists, and others commonly called it, no thought of the Medical Center as it now exists was in their mind. The members of the board of health showed immediate interest in this building, especially Dr. Henry Petersen and Dr. E. W. Bertner. Both mentioned it many times when they appeared publicly to talk about the health needs of Houston. As members of the board of health, we were all asked many times to speak before public gatherings. A school of public health was included with the other schools— medicine, dentistry, and nursing along with medical, dental, and nursing technology in the plans for the Memorial Center for Health Education. This was a good talking point for the members of the board of health when they gave public health lectures.

A complete hospital and clinic occupied the upper floors of the building. The library and administrative offices were located on the two floors of the extended tower. Dr. Petersen always described the plan for the total use of the building since he wanted his listeners to understand the importance of the interrelationships that could be developed between the professions

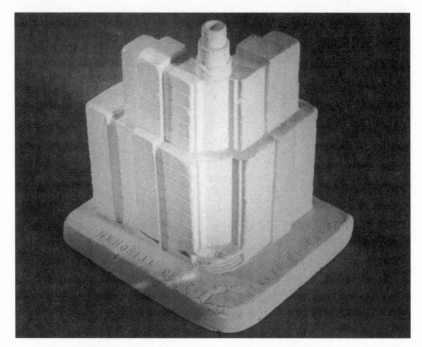

Plaster model of Memorial Center for Health Education.

and the ancillary groups. He emphasized the inadequacy of the present scattering of the schools over an entire university campus. Meanwhile, others also promoted the idea.

Mrs. Birath talked to the Rotary Anns at one of their luncheons in early 1939. These ladies immediately became interested in the building. At the time the Rotary Anns were seeking a project that they could support that they felt was a real need in Houston. At a later meeting of the Rotary Anns, I discussed with them the idea of a dental health foundation. This was an idea I had proposed earlier to the board of the newly established Ripley Foundation. One of the treatment services to be provided in the dental health building, one in which I believed that the Rotary Anns might be interested, was an "orthodontia clinic." This did appeal to the Rotary Anns, and they adopted it as a project. The program was started immediately in the Texas Dental College. Later, it was transferred to a clinic provided in the Ripley House, which was supported by the Ripley Foundation.

The Memorial Center for Health Education had impressed many dentists. At the annual meeting of the dental college alumni association in 1939,

Dr. Emil Tejml, president of the association, proposed that the alumni association actively support the idea for a Memorial Center for Health Education by making contact with citizens in their community. He informed the alumni members present at the meeting that the Memorial Center for Health Education was to be an endowed institution. Therefore, it was necessary that some foundation become interested in the project. Dr. Tejml had several large Texas foundations in mind.

We continued to have monthly meetings of the dental college board of trustees. They were time consuming, yet important. I felt it was necessary that members of the board, the faculty, the employees, and the students were kept informed about all activities of the college, as well as the actions we were required to take to meet the obligations of the college. Mrs. Birath and I appreciated the strong interest the trustees showed in the detailed reports we made. She remarked to me many times about the sacrifice of time—both days and evenings—the members made for the trustee meetings or when we needed their personal support. Dr. Finis M. Hight, president of the board of trustees, and many other trustees gave not only their time, but also helped finance many projects that could not be carried forward without their help. All of them were devoted teachers as well. I recall that one year Dr. Hight

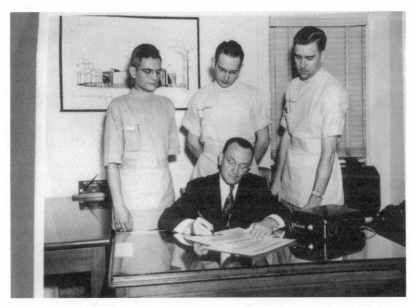

Elliott as dean of Texas Dental College, signing diplomas in his office, early 1950s.

held two- and three-hour evening sessions for the senior class. He was giving a special clinic course that used actual patients and was devoting almost all of his evenings to dental college projects. Suddenly and sadly, his wise counsel and guidance ended. Dr. Hight died an untimely death on November 2, 1939. Ann and I had lost one of our very close and warm friends.

At the board meeting on December 12, 1939, Dr. Judson L. Taylor was elected as a member of the board. He was to take the place of Dr. Hight. The trustees again asked Dr. Walter Scherer to serve as president. At this meeting I reported to the board my growing friendship with the new dean of the Medical Branch of the University of Texas. Dr. George Bethel, the former dean of the Medical Branch, died in 1935, and Dr. W. S. Carter, who had served as dean of the Medical Branch from 1903 to 1922, returned to the Medical Branch to serve again as interim dean until a new dean was appointed. He resigned when Dr. John Spies arrived in the fall of 1939.

John Spies was the brother of Dr. Tom Spies, a noted medical researcher in the field of nutrition. I had discussed with Dr. Bethel the possibility of the dental school becoming a part of the university early in 1935. Dr. Bethel did not mention the part he had played in 1931 when the Medical Branch had attempted to establish a dental school in Galveston. I did not mention this incident to him, either. I did not visit Galveston again to talk with Dr. Carter. Both Drs. Carter and Bethel had served as deans through the period when the Medical Branch had made unsuccessful attempts to establish a dental school in Galveston. As I related this information to the board, I noticed that they were quite interested. I informed the board that Dr. Spies had shown interest in the Texas Dental College's desire to become a part of the University of Texas. At this meeting I was authorized to continue my discussions with Dr. Spies and to proceed with whatever action was necessary to increase Dr. Spies's interest in our college. Through the years Dr. Spies and I became warm friends. We worked together for the aims that he and I envisioned. We agreed that the Medical Branch's budget should be given first consideration by the legislature [in 1941] since at the time the Council on Medical Education was criticizing the branch concerning improvements that were needed for the school. Dr. Spies was to request a budget that reflected a tremendous increase over the previous year.[1]

It was clear that it was not the time to propose a dental branch of the University of Texas. I was sure that had we done so, it would have resulted in another failure. I believed that we would need more time to get members of the legislature and their constituents fully informed of the need for a state dental college as a part of the University of Texas. Also, I did not wish to lose

Dr. Spies's help. I knew that we must not fail again or we would no longer exist. Dr. Spies was pleased that I agreed with him that the dental college should wait until the next session of the legislature before it presented its plan to become a part of the university. He told me he would be with us all the way *if* his budget request was approved. Otherwise, he would resign. I did all that I could to help him get approval of his budget request [and both bills passed in 1941].

I saw Dr. Spies frequently. My appointment as a lecturer in stomatology to the senior class of the medical school required that I make weekly trips to Galveston. After my lectures Dr. Spies always invited me to visit with him. While we discussed many topics, Dr. Spies's plan for improving the educational facilities of the Medical Branch was the most interesting to me. Many of Dr. Spies's ideas could be used for the dental college. Dr. Spies also discussed a dental education plan that he had developed in China when he was with the Rockefeller Foundation. It was from this dentistry connection that he had become interested in our dental college in Houston.

Early in 1940, Dr. Spies began to make contact with county medical societies throughout the state. The members of the societies introduced him to many of the prominent citizens in their communities. Dr. Spies always frankly discussed the large budget request that he would make of the legislature in 1941. During his visits to various county societies, he also made it a point to become acquainted with members of the legislature in that district. Dr. Spies's appropriation bill was in the hopper early in the session of the 1941 legislature. News accounts, which appeared in local newspapers following an address by Dr. Spies, informed the public about the medical school's needs. Many people were disturbed when they read Dr. Spies's comments concerning the attitude of the Council on Medical Education. Dr. Spies was in Austin at the time his bill was introduced. A short time after his arrival, Arthur Cato, a House member from Weatherford, introduced himself to Dr. Spies and asked for Spies's support for his cancer hospital bill. Dr. Spies was immediately interested in Cato's bill. This was a familiar project to him since he had worked on a cancer hospital program in India. He recognized that the Cato bill would be a tremendous help to him. He informed Mr. Cato of his own bill and told him that they should work closely together. Representative Cato and Dr. Spies became close working partners.[2]

On those occasions that I was required to go to Austin during the legislative session, I visited with Dr. Spies. I listened with interest to his explanations how he was proceeding to get a favorable reaction from the legislature. He reported several of the conversations that he had with legislators to me. Our conversations were informative, because I could later use many of the activities that Dr. Spies was developing. It was at one of my meetings with Dr. Spies that I had the opportunity to meet Arthur Cato. At this time I learned the nature of Cato's bill for creating cancer hospitals in Texas. It was while the legislature was in session that a story about the M. D. Anderson Foundation appeared in the newspaper. Monroe D. Anderson, a co-founder of Anderson, Clayton & Co., had died August 6, 1939. The story announced that Mr. Anderson had established a foundation in his name. The article stated that Mr. Anderson desired to have the proceeds of his estate be used for broad purposes for the good of the people of Texas. The article also announced the names of the members of the board of trustees of the Anderson Foundation. I read the article with considerable interest, because this foundation might be interested in supporting the Memorial Center for Health Education.[3]

Colonel William B. Bates was chairman of the board of the new foundation. The other members were John Freeman and Horace Wilkins. The interest that Colonel Bates had shown in the dental college in 1931 led me to believe that he might be interested in the plan for the Memorial Center for Health Education. I explained this plan to Dr. Spies and he showed some interest in it. However, he suggested that it should be the University of Texas Center in Houston. This suggestion pleased me because Dr. Spies pointed out that the budget for such an operation would be so large that it would require state support. Dr. Spies telephoned me the next day after the article about M. D. Anderson appeared in the paper. He asked me if I knew Colonel Bates, the chairman of the foundation board. I told him that I was acquainted with Colonel Bates, that he had shown considerable interest in the University of Texas, and that he had been quite interested in the welfare of the Texas Dental College. It was later that Dr. Spies was to visit with Colonel Bates at his home in Houston. At the time, I did not know of the visit. I learned later that Colonel Bates had expressed interest in the cancer hospital, but told Dr. Spies that a such hospital belonged in a city larger than Galveston.

Nothing that Colonel Bates could have said could have pleased Dr. Spies anymore than this remark. Dr. Spies readily agreed with Colonel Bates. He told him that if the board saw fit to help build the hospital that he saw no problem in trying to locate the hospital in Houston. No definite plans had been made as to where it would be located, yet. It was just a few days later that the Anderson Foundation made an announcement that a grant of $500,000 would be made to the University of Texas for the construction of a cancer hospital, provided that it was built in Houston. Now Dr. Spies and Representative Cato had a real offer to make to the legislature. The Memorial Center for Health Education, as such, was shelved by the dental college. A few days after this announcement appeared in the newspapers, Dr. Spies called me and asked if I were coming to Austin soon. I had planned to be in Austin the following day. I first called on Carl Hardin, a practicing attorney in Austin, who also served as the attorney and legislative representative both for the State Board of Dental Examiners and the Texas State Dental Society. I told Mr. Hardin that I was in Austin to meet with Dr. Spies for lunch. But, before doing so, I wanted to discuss with him some of my previous conversations with Dr. Spies concerning the plans to make the Texas Dental College a branch of the University of Texas. I informed Carl Hardin that Dr. Spies had agreed to help us all that he could. However, I explained to Hardin that Dr. Spies did not wish for us to make any move during the 1941 session, as he did not want anything to interfere with his budget request for the Medical Branch. I told Hardin that I agreed with Dr. Spies that we should wait.

I asked Mr. Hardin if it were possible for him to assist us in our approach to the legislature. He asked me to assemble some material for him so that he could discuss it with the members of the State Board of Dental Examiners and the officers of the Texas State Dental Society. It was Hardin's opinion that both of these bodies should be informed fully of our plan and that they should actively support the plan that was developed. He said that he should devote most of his time now and during the legislative session of 1943 to the dental college bill. After my conversation with Carl Hardin, I returned to the hotel for the luncheon with Dr. Spies. After lunch we went to his room and continued our discussion. During our conversation, Dr. Spies abruptly stopped the discussion about the legislative session and said that he wanted to discuss with me, confidentially, another matter concerning the Medical Branch and the dental school. He made it a point to emphasize that I must not discuss this matter with others. He told me that when he had learned that the cancer hospital bill would be supported by the Anderson Foundation, that the idea came to him that he would concentrate on developing plans for the Houston part of the program if the bill were approved.

Spies said that he would actively engage in getting support for the approval of the dental school as a branch of the university. Since the cancer hospital was to be built in Houston he wanted the dental school also to continue operating in Houston. Here he sprung his confidential surprise. It was his plan to use these two institutions that were planned for Houston as a springboard for moving the Medical Branch from Galveston to Houston. He said that this would require considerable time and that there would be no announcement made of such a plan. His first move was to start a clinic center in Houston as a unit of the Medical Branch. The purpose of the clinic would be to provide facilities for improved education of the medical students. He believed that it could become a part of the hospital training program for the medical students. He would appoint a part-time faculty made up from the staffs of the various hospitals in Houston, especially Jefferson Davis Hospital.

At the closing hours of the legislature, both budget requests for the Medical Branch and the Cato bill passed the House and the Senate. Now Dr. Spies could rapidly proceed with the plans he had in mind. It was time now for us at the dental college to pull out all the stops and devote our full energies toward the 1943 legislative session. Following adjournment of the 1941 legislative session, we immediately stepped up our public information program at the dental college. I arranged meetings with Mr. Blanton, executive vice president of the chamber of commerce; Mr. Bryan, president of the Second National Bank board; all members of the board of health, officers of the medical society; the Houston District Dental Society; and the state dental association.

I arranged an appointment with Dr. Homer Rainey, president of the university, to discuss the possibility of a dental college for the university. He expressed no opinion, but said he would discuss the idea with other university officials. I talked with the Houston member of the board of regents. He was quite interested and told me that he would recommend the idea to other members of the board who he thought would be receptive to the proposal, but that he would not ask for formal approval at this time.

Several of the groups that I had contacted appointed special committees to work with our faculty members, students, and personnel. Some developed excellent ideas that would help the cause. Mrs. Birath, Miss Cline (my secretary), and I were assembling facts and statistics that would serve to compare the inadequate dental educational facilities in Texas with other state dental schools that had university affiliations. The material was included in the brochures that were prepared for public dental schools. One day, a student brought an amusing illustration to me that made this comparison in a graphic manner. We used it as a cover page for one of the circulars that was prepared for statewide distribution.

One day I was laying sewer tile to drain our driveway, when I saw Ann running toward me. Her face was ashen. She started crying as she ran toward me—the Japanese had bombed Pearl Harbor! I was astounded. Why? We knew nothing about any difficulty with Japan. I could hardly comprehend the horror of this as she continued to relate to me the extent of the attack. It was Sunday, December 7, 1941. At once the vision of 1918 flashed into my mind. What would happen? Would the government take the same action now as they had in World War I? Would our plan for a state school be dashed to the ground? Would the school be forced to close because of financial difficulties caused by a reduced enrollment? The news about the war was frightening.

At the dental college, students were concerned about their education. Both students and faculty in the reserve forces were called into service immediately. Other patriotic students wanted to enlist also. We asked both students and faculty members to wait for government action before doing so. The students and faculty in Kansas City had a similar reaction in 1918. I reminded the faculty members and students that a large number of trained professionals would be in demand for medical and dental services. It was necessary that the country's dental and medical colleges make provisions to provide the armed forces the physicians and dentists they needed.[4]

Within a short time, I was asked to serve on evaluation boards that were to select student "pre-meds" or "pre-dents" that had been drafted by the army or the navy. Those that were approved by the board would be deferred until graduation. This proved to be a most difficult and trying assignment. Medical and dental students who were in college at the time were ordered to remain in college. They would not be permitted to enter the armed services. It was the responsibility of presidents and deans of universities and colleges to classify faculty members whom they believed were essential for the education of students, even though some of them wanted to resign and go into service. It was not long until we were reorganizing the teaching program for a three-year program to replace the normal four-year plan that was in operation. This meant a twelve-month curriculum. I had experience with this procedure since the same plan had been followed during World War I.

The public drive [to affiliate with the University of Texas] began early in 1942 and swept the state in a surprisingly short time. We received letter after letter from citizens from every part of the state pledging their support. When the legislative session began in January, 1943, I was tremendously encouraged by the favorable attitude that had been shown by legislators from almost every section of the state.

One day, Dr. Scherer, president of the board of trustees of the dental college, suggested that he and I meet with Col. W. B. Bates, chairman of the

Anderson Foundation, who was also a patient of Dr. Scherer's. We would ask him to advise us on how we should present our case to the committee when we were called to make our presentation. Dr. Scherer did not want us to make any errors when we appeared before the committee. He remembered that Colonel Bates had made the presentation for the dental school at the committee hearing in 1931. We had made it clear in all of the material that we had prepared that the Texas Dental College would close if our bill passed. Also, all of the property and assets of the Texas Dental College would be given to the university without any strings attached and the board of regents would be free to locate the dental school wherever they wished. When Colonel Bates heard this, he was pleased. He remembered that this had not been made clear in 1931, and that it was, in his opinion, the reason that the dental school bill did not pass at that time. Colonel Bates told Dr. Scherer that he would give some thought on how we should proceed and call Dr. Scherer later. As we expressed our appreciation for his time and walked toward the door, Colonel Bates stopped us, remarking that he was very pleased with the operation of the dental school during the past few years. He felt that we would have little difficulty in convincing the legislators that a university school was needed. Then, he made a remark that overwhelmed both Dr. Scherer and me. He said to Dr. Scherer, "I believe the Anderson Foundation may want to help. Possibly we could make a grant of $500,000 to the university for the purpose of establishing a dental school. Of course," he said, "I will need to discuss this idea with the other trustees of the foundation." We were both speechless at first. Then Dr. Scherer expressed our sincere appreciation. I could only say, "Thank you, Colonel Bates," and we left. It was but a few days later that we read in the papers that this grant would be made to the University of Texas if the pending bill for the dental school were passed.

During 1942, we continued the activities that were underway in preparation for the 1943 legislative session, burning the midnight oil. War demands called for more professionals in all fields. It was necessary for me to meet with the university officials and legislators, as well as the service command officers. We were pleased with the favorable attitude of all those whom we discussed our university plans with.

The newspapers and radios reported constantly on the medical needs of the services. This, though sad, helped us in our legislative endeavors. Casualties were mounting. Thousands of soldiers were being wounded. Head, face, and mouth injuries far exceeded those of World War I. Dentists and oral surgeons were badly needed. Hundreds of physician and dentist offices were being closed because the doctors were on their way to war as volunteers. Through these hectic days, Dr. Spies and I met occasionally to discuss our plans. He was busily engaged in war activities at the Medical Branch and had little time to work with us on the dental school program. I was thrown into contact with Dr. Bailey Calvin, assistant dean of the Medical Branch, and Dr. Don Slaughter, dean of the Southwestern Medical College in Dallas. Often, we were together on the selection boards of the army and navy.

My appointment as a lecturer in stomatology at the Medical Branch early in December, 1938, placed me in an awkward position. It seems that almost immediately after Dr. Spies had been appointed dean of the Medical Branch in the fall of 1938, disagreements began developing between him and some members of the faculty, but I did not know of this at the time. Dr. Edward Randall of Galveston, a member of the Board of Regents, previously had a long association with the faculty, causing him to sympathize with their grievances. At a meeting of the board of regents in late October, 1939, Dr. Randall presented the matter of these disagreements to the board. It appears that the board did not take the action that Dr. Randall wanted. Consequently, Dr. Randall resigned from the board of regents early in 1940 and immediately issued a quite derogatory public statement to Dr. Spies.

An excerpt from this statement explains the tenor of the release: "Dr. Spies, although an American and native-born Texan, in my opinion, employs totalitarian methods." Rather explosive! From here on I was on pins and needles. However, this statement seemingly had no effect on the legislators since Dr. Spies's budget request was approved. It tripled the previous appropriation! The legislature appropriated $1,350,000 for the Medical Branch and $500,000 for the cancer research hospital.

The board of regents found themselves besieged with complaints from the faculty members of the Medical Branch, from many Galvestonians, and from board members of a foundation in Galveston about Dr. Spies. This barrage of complaints resulted in Spies's dismissal. Just two weeks later, the board of regents reversed this action and re-appointed him dean for an additional two years. Following this, Dr. Spies took a vacation. While he was away, a special faculty committee presented a petition to President Rainey. Every member of the faculty had signed it. Rainey took no action since the board of regents had just re-appointed Dr. Spies for two more years.

Dr. Rainey was now further involved in difficulties with the Medical Branch faculty. We at the dental college assumed the attitude of the three monkeys—hear no evil, see no evil, speak no evil. It was a trying situation for us. I did not want to offend Dr. Spies by resigning my lectureship; neither did I want to antagonize members of the faculty of the Medical Branch. The faculty committee decided to move in a different direction. They raised many serious charges against Dr. Spies. They discussed the items in the appropriation bill, which they felt were allocating funds in the wrong direction. One of the items they mentioned was that eleven thousand dollars had been appropriated for the establishment of a department of stomatology and dentistry at the medical school. This was the first I had heard of this item on Dr. Spies's budget. I was puzzled and tried to conjecture just what purpose Dr. Spies had in mind for establishing such a department at the Medical Branch. I did not have the opportunity to discuss this with Dr. Spies before he was dismissed as dean of the Medical Branch in June, 1942.

It was very soon after I had begun my trips to Galveston, sometime in the early spring of 1942, that I learned of the seriousness of the dissention that had developed between Dr. Spies and the faculty. Dr. D. Bailey Calvin, who had taught physiological chemistry at Yale University and later at the University of Missouri, had joined the faculty at the Medical Branch in 1937. I met Dr. Calvin when he was appointed associate dean in 1942. Previously, however, Dr. Calvin and I had become warm friends while working together on the selection committee of the army and navy. It was during these committee meetings that I learned the serious situation that existed in Galveston. Dr. Calvin steered me away from many of the dangerous shoals. His position made it necessary for him to be with Dr. Spies frequently. They occupied adjoining offices. Naturally, Dr. Calvin and I were both concerned about the unfortunate developments at the Medical Branch, but as administrators we recognized that Dr. Spies was in an untenable position, and to us it seemed that he rather enjoyed it. We learned very early that we were to listen, not advise.

I met with Dr. Rainey frequently in 1942. This was possible because I was attending state board of health meetings. My purpose was to keep Dr. Rainey informed of our plans as they related to the approaching legislative session. He suggested the type of material we should submit to the board of regents when Dr. Scherer transferred the Texas Dental College properties and assets to the university. During these visits to Austin, I became acquainted with many members of the legislature in my capacity as a state board of health member. Our board appeared many times before committee meetings. Also, I had become acquainted with members of the board of regents through the Houston member at the time. Carl Hardin made it a point that I meet other state officers, including the governor. These contacts would serve us well at the time our bill was being considered by the legislature. It was on one of my trips to Austin that I learned, through an *Austin American-Statesman* headline, that Dr. Spies had been fired. I was quite upset because I feared that the new administrator appointed at the Medical Branch might hamper our legislative effort. My anxiety abated when I later learned that the committee had selected Dr. Titus Harris to serve as acting dean until a new administrative officer was appointed.[5]

I met Dr. Spies in the hotel lobby on the day that he received the news. He was on his way back to Galveston. He seemed quite depressed, but he smiled as he came toward me and said, "I have been fired." I expressed my regret and told him I would miss him very much. I also told him that this action would grieve both Ann and me. I was not to see him again until much later.

During this period, the [compressed] three-year teaching program had been operating smoothly. However, it was a tiring situation for the faculty. They had very little rest during the year since only three weeks could be allowed for vacation and lecture preparation for the next session. I continued some of my civic activities, but many had been discontinued because of the war. Most of the organizations that continued were devoting their energies to war projects.

Shortly after Dr. Spies's dismissal, Dr. Judson Taylor called me and asked that we have lunch together. During the luncheon he told me the purpose of his call had to do with the cancer hospital. He was concerned that unless some move was made quickly, someone might be appointed acting director that would not be suitable for our plans in Houston. He suggested that Dr. Ernst William Bertner serve as acting director for the cancer hospital until a permanent director was appointed, which, he thought, would require quite some time. He had shared this idea with Dr. Bertner already and learned that Bertner was agreeable but somewhat reluctant to accept since he was overwhelmed with work. Dr. Taylor asked me to recommend Dr. Bertner to Dr. Rainey for this appointment, which I did. Dr. Rainey asked me several questions and then told me that he would recommend the appointment of Dr. Bertner to the board of regents.

I informed Dr. Taylor of my conversation with Dr. Rainey. I did not know at the time that Dr. Taylor had also discussed this idea with one of the members of the executive committee of the chamber of commerce. They, too, recommended Dr. Bertner. The board of regents appointed him as acting director of the cancer hospital at the July meeting in 1942. It was announced in the press on August 1. At the time that Dr. Bertner accepted the appointment, he declined the salary of ten thousand dollars that the board offered to him. He told the chairman of the board of regents that he would prefer that they apply this amount to the budget for the cancer hospital. Dr. Taylor and I were well pleased. Dr. Bertner and I became even more closely associated as working partners in our development of plans for the university projects, which then were only the dental branch and the cancer hospital. Dr. Spies had had little opportunity to develop plans for the cancer hospital because of the difficulty he was having with the faculty, and also because the faculty of the Medical Branch had no time to devote to the cancer hospital because of the war.

After it was announced in August, 1942, that Dr. Bertner had been appointed as acting director of the cancer hospital, we were together more frequently. His appointment as an official of the university preceded my own official relationship to the university. Dr. Bertner made rapid progress in developing plans for the cancer hospital. The Anderson Foundation acquired the Baker Estate on Baldwin Street. This property would serve as temporary quarters for the cancer hospital of the University of Texas [non-war related construction was prohibited until after the war]. Dr. Bertner employed architects to develop plans for a clinic building, which would adjoin the main house. The main house was converted to an office and staff building. The basement of the main house was converted to temporary quarters for the x-ray equipment.

Dr. Bertner asked that I study the floor plans for the temporary clinic building and make suggestions for any changes I thought necessary. I made several minor suggestions, including to enlarge the clinic reception room. This was done; however, it proved entirely inadequate. Several faculty members and business personnel from the Medical Branch were "loaned" to the cancer hospital by Dr. Leake. At the time, both the cancer hospital and the medical school were under his jurisdiction. The Baker Property stables were remodeled for use as research laboratories and the faculty members from Galveston directed the planning for these laboratories. Dr. Fritz Schlenk was the biochemist, and Dr. C. P. Coogle also occupied one of the laboratories.[6]

January, 1943, arrived and House Bill 279 and a companion bill in the Senate were introduced early in the session. Carl Hardin and I were together constantly. I spent every moment in Austin when it was not necessary for me to be elsewhere. The days seemed to me to pass ever so slowly. When would the dental school bill be brought to the floor of the House? Both the Senate and House committees had approved it. Hardin and I waited in the gallery day after day. We met with legislators and senators at lunch. We talked with dentists on every occasion and asked them to contact their patients and have the patients write to their senator or legislator. Many of them came to Austin in support of the dental school bill. Still we waited. Each day, as we sat in the gallery, we would become alert every time the gavel sounded and a new bill was called, only to be disappointed when it was not our bill. The session was nearing the end.

One day, late in the session, Carl Hardin and I went to lunch. We had always returned promptly to the House gallery after lunch so that we would not miss the call to order, but on this day we were a little late. To our surprise, when we returned the House was already in session. While we waited to learn the title of the bill that was being considered, someone tapped me on the shoulder. It was a dentist friend of mine. He spoke one word: "Congratulations!" Carl and I were startled. We had missed the vote that we had been waiting for so many days, weeks, and months! The bill had passed within the first few minutes after the gavel had sounded. My friend informed us that only two dissenting votes were cast.

Though chagrined that we had missed the exciting moments of roll call, Carl and I were walking on a cloud. We were to exchange our seats in the House gallery for seats in the Senate. During the long period it had taken to reach this point, other events had happened. President Rainey was becoming more and more involved in confrontations with the board of regents. I had a rebound from one of the president's preceding difficulties with a Senator Moore from Harris County. This occurred before our bill was brought to the floor of the Senate. I was in the Senate one day when a page came to me and informed me that Senator Moore wished to see me. When I entered Moore's office, I saw that he was angry. He had just seen the bill as it had come from the House. He informed me that he was going to change the bill as it had been passed by the House and refer it back to committee. This blunt statement left me almost speechless.

I asked Senator Moore what was wrong with the bill as it was passed by the House. He told me in language that need not be repeated and that displayed his dislike for President Rainey. He said that he would not allow me, as dean of the college and for whom he had great respect (his words), to report to the president of the university as the House bill stipulated. He said that he was going to strike this clause from the bill and that he would substitute a clause that required me to report to the board of regents rather than the president. He changed the bill in this manner. Later, in a Senate committee meeting, he conceded that it was not an important matter. The bill was left as it was and returned to the Senate. Carl and I breathed a sigh of relief. I learned later what had caused Senator Moore to dislike President Rainey. In addition to the ongoing controversy with the board of regents, there also was the matter of a book that had been published and placed in the university library, which the senator wanted removed. However, President Rainey refused to remove the book. This episode was only one of the many which had kept me in a state of anxiety from late 1940 until House Bill 279 became law in 1943.[7]

On June 26, 1943, a news story released by the board of regents announced the appointment of the first clinical staff of the cancer hospital, all of whom were prominent physicians and surgeons in Houston. Those named were Joe B. Foster, John H. Foster, E. L. Goar, Herbert T. Hayes, Robert A. Johnston, Ben Weems Turner, James Greenwood, C. M. Griswold, M. D. Levy, David Greer, Judson Taylor, John H. Poster, E. W. Bertner, and me, Frederick C. Elliot. Dr. Bertner had selected the staff and recommended them to the board of regents. It was not until March 1, 1944, that the first patients arrived at the doors of the new outpatient department. Anna Hanselman, who had worked for Dr. Bertner, was the first staff nurse and was in charge of the admission of patients. John Musgrove served as business manager of the cancer hospital, on "loan" from the Medical Branch. Dr. Bertner, as chief of services in his field at Hermann Hospital, had contracted with the hospital for the use of beds, which were to be reserved for the cancer hospital. I attended several of the cancer hospital's staff conferences for preoperative case reports. I found these sessions informative. They gave me a closer view of the tremendous task that confronted Dr. Bertner and his staff. The unknowns seemed to be unlimited. The new director, when he came, was to have an awesome and insurmountable task.[8]

Full days and almost full nights of activities and excitement were ahead for Dr. Bertner and me. We were both moving towards realizing an organized plan for a university medical center in Houston. At the same time, Dr. Bertner continued a very busy schedule with his practice and his duties as acting director of the cancer hospital. I continued with the health committee and community activities, as well as meeting nightly with the faculty to discuss the development of plans for the programs for our new university dental branch in the years to come. The faculty continued to have full days of school activity. Those of us who later had the opportunity to discuss these early years wonder how we did it at all. Dr. Bertner and I continued to work on plans for the University of Texas institutions to be located in Houston. Time passed quickly. The dental branch of the university was given more and more attention by the press and by the public. Dr. Bertner and I talked before many groups concerning the possibilities and plans for the university institutions in Houston. Members of the board of trustees of the Anderson Foundation devoted considerable time in discussions with university officials and with Dr. Leake, Dr. Bertner, and myself concerning the developing plans.

In May, 1943, Dr. Rainey was in Houston to meet with members of the Anderson Foundation Board of Trustees and with Dr. Bertner and me to talk about actions taken by the university board of regents and himself. On the morning of May 5, 1943, the *Houston Post* reported on Dr. Rainey's discussion, quoting one statement of significant importance as far as the university and medical center relationships were concerned. Rainey's statement was: "The University of Texas will have supervision over the entire center." Yet, on May 8, 1943, just three days later, it was announced that Baylor University and the Anderson Foundation had reached an agreement whereby Baylor Medical College and Baylor Dental College would be moved to Houston. Dr. Bertner and I were taken by surprise since we had not known of this action until we read of it in the morning paper. We learned later that the reason for this action was that the Anderson Foundation had quietly studied the possibility of moving the Medical Branch of the University of Texas to Houston and found that it was most unlikely that this move could ever be made. They desired for a medical school to be located in the center that was being planned. Now, Dr. Bertner and I had to develop plans to include two new schools in the medical center. Likewise, the program's orientation would need to be changed. Baylor University decided later not to move the dental college to Houston. This was a wise decision, since today Baylor College of Dentistry is one of the leading dental colleges in the United States.

Dr. Chauncey Leake was fast becoming well known as the president for medical affairs of the University of Texas. Since his arrival in September, 1942, he had skillfully developed an excellent relationship with all whom he was associated. His approach to the problems that confronted him was one of graciousness, hospitality, and candor. His manner was gentle, but frank. He met with faculty members individually as well as collectively. Past conditions were discussed so that they could be forgotten. The medical school moved into a positive position everyone welcomed and admired. Dr. Bertner and I, like his faculty, admired and respected Dr. Leake. We met with him frequently during the early part of 1943 to discuss the Houston affairs and the development of plans for the overall university campus in Houston. Dr. Leake contributed many ideas and discussed other institutions that should be a part of the overall health education program in Houston. Among these were the Institute of Gerontology, the Institute of Geographic Medicine, a library and historical institute, and several others. He enthusiastically supported the idea for a school of public health. He suggested that the Texas A&M college should be included in the plans for the development of the public health school and should work with the new public health facility. He talked at length about the need for the development of an outstanding library in Houston and stated that it should be of such quality as to challenge the nation. His enthusiasm was catching. He made public announcements of every intention he might have to gain numerous news interviews. President Rainey supported Leake in his suggestions.

Dr. Bertner and I were now engaged in a challenge that caused us both to double our energies, if that were possible. While not discussing it, we felt that some time soon the Medical Branch would develop a program of health education in Houston, yet it was not to be solely a University of Texas health center. Dr. Bertner made many trips to various centers throughout the United States. He was especially impressed by the Institute of Rehabilitative Medicine of New York University Medical Center, directed by Dr. Howard A. Rusk. Dr. Bertner liked the institute's plan so well that he invited Dr. Rusk to visit Houston and discuss it at a special public meeting. Dr. Rusk told Dr. Bertner in New York that he felt the development of a medical center without an institute for rehabilitation would be a serious mistake. All of these announcements excited us at the dental college. We were becoming more and more enthusiastic and proud that we would become a part of this huge total program.

I should go back and explain in more detail the reasons why the Anderson Foundation made the decision to bring Baylor University College of Medicine to Houston. The idea that Dr. Spies had quietly discussed with me early in 1941, which was to move the Medical Branch from Galveston to Houston, was now an open discussion among many people throughout Texas. Dr. Spies had no doubt discussed it with some of the faculty members whom he had brought to Galveston. Many of these younger faculty were quite interested in making the move for the same reasons as Dr. Spies. During that time the idea of the move was brought to the attention of the legislature, possibly in 1941. Dr. Raymond Gregory, who was on the faculty of the Medical Branch, was asked to appear before a legislative committee to discuss the proposal in a logical and reasonable manner. Dr. Gregory made no recommendations, leaving the question open for the legislature to decide.

During this period, Baylor University College of Medicine was having a considerable amount of discussion with members of the medical profession in Dallas about a move on foot to establish a new school of medicine there. These discussions caused the board of trustees of Baylor University to decide that the Baylor Medical College should be moved away from Dallas. No action was taken by the Texas legislature to move the medical college from Galveston, so one of the members of the Baylor board of trustees contacted a member of the Anderson Foundation board and made inquiries concerning the possibility of moving Baylor University College of Medicine to Houston. This move was made, but at the time our dental college was not a part of the University of Texas. Dr. Bertner and I continued to discuss the manner in which a coordinated medical center could be developed. We decided it best to wait until Baylor College of Medicine was operating in Houston before going too far with discussions of coordinating Baylor and the University of Texas in a total medical center program. Yet, we did decide that we should develop a plan that could be given careful study so that, at the proper time, we could submit a proposal that was workable.

Dr. Bertner asked me to prepare a draft of such a plan for our discussions. After I had developed the plan I took it to Dr. Bertner. He discussed our ideas with John Freeman, a trustee of the Anderson Foundation. After listening to Dr. Bertner, Freeman suggested that it was his idea that the medical center should be an independent one. Freeman had just returned from a trip east and had conceived an idea for a center from his visits to other independently organized medical educational centers. He was of the opinion that an independent organization would facilitate the inclusion of other health education and research institutions in the medical center. All of us thought this idea was excellent. John Freeman suggested the name, and the "Texas Medical Center" was finally on its way to becoming a reality.

Some time later, the first meeting of a group suggested by Dr. Bertner was held to select those who would be invited to serve as members of the board of trustees of the Texas Medical Center. During this time the Anderson Foundation had been seeking a possible location for the medical center and decided that the tract just south of Hermann Hospital would be an ideal location. The land contained about 134 acres and had been given to the city of Houston by Mr. Will Hogg for park purposes. The Anderson Foundation trustees met with city officials and learned that although they were enthusiastic about the transaction, the voters of Houston first must approve it. At the special election called for this purpose on December 14, 1943, the public voted, approving the project, and the city sold the land to the Anderson

Foundation. The Anderson Foundation employed H. A. Kipp, who had developed the River Oaks subdivision, to develop the tract for the Texas Medical Center.

The Medical Center had not yet been officially organized and issued a charter. The war was still on and because of it, it was not possible to obtain new members for our faculty. Our clinical staff was overworked. During this period we were developing and experimenting with new ideas as they related to the plans for teaching in our new building. We discussed these plans with Dr. Leake, who was quite interested in our plans for the new building. He told me about an innovative plan for laboratory teaching. He developed the plan while he was a faculty member at the University of Wisconsin, but his plan was not used there. He had published an article describing the plan and said that he would mail me a reprint. It described in detail Dr. Leake's laboratory plan that he had developed. Our faculty became so interested in this teaching plan that we had a similar model laboratory constructed. He had suggested twelve students in each laboratory. We reduced the number to four because we planned to include the dental science courses, as well as the basic science courses. We also gave consideration to clinical teaching. Our unit plan included a separate office for each student. This was innovative because now the student was responsible for his own learning. It was the student's responsibility to care for both the basic science laboratory and the clinic cubicle that was assigned to him. Each student would be required to maintain the equipment, as well as complete the janitorial service required for both units. This plan proved to be the forerunner of an educational plan used by many other colleges in the United States. It has been modified and improved, yet the basic idea remains the same. The philosophy behind the unit method was to make the student responsible for his own learning. Naturally, the entire curriculum would need to be revised. Many innovative ideas that each faculty member developed became a part of the plan. Departments were reorganized and teaching methods were changed. Not all of these changes met the approval of some of the faculty members who saw little need for change—old shoes were more comfortable.

Plans for our relationship with Baylor University College of Medicine were developing. The remodeling of the old Sears building, which would provide temporary facilities for Baylor University College of Medicine, was completed and they moved to Houston in May, 1943. The faculty and staff of the Baylor College of Medicine found that the move from Dallas was not one to soon be forgotten. They had a very short time to make the move because of the war. Soon after they were settled in their new quarters, I had the opportunity to visit with Dr. Walter Moursund, the dean of the college. On one of my visits with Dr. Moursund, I asked him if there were a possibility that some of his faculty members might be willing to teach basic science courses in the dental school. He felt that this could be arranged. Four faculty members of the medical school agreed to serve as instructors in those departments for which we did not have full-time instructors.

It was during the first part of the year that Dr. Bertner announced the members of the first staff of the cancer hospital. The officers of the Chamber of Commerce, elated over our success in Austin, honored me with a dinner. I responded by reminding them that the Chamber of Commerce and the people of Houston were responsible for our success.

Also in June, Margaret Jones graduated from the dental college. During the summer session of Miss Jones's junior year, she and a senior dental student were sailing with Dr. Ellen Wellensiek, a faculty member of the dental school. They sailed to a favorite swimming hole and began lowering the sail as they approached the swimming area. Miss Jones and her escort jumped out to swim. As they played in the water, Miss Jones grabbed the mast-stay. Her escort surfaced and playfully seized Miss Jones just below the shoulders. At that very moment, the steel mast-stay contacted a high voltage line. Miss Jones lost both her arms and her friend died in this split-second accident. It was a terrible tragedy for the dental college. When Miss Jones recovered, we decided that she should graduate with her class. Dr. Jones completed her master's degree in public health at the University of Michigan and later joined the faculty of Meharry Medical College in Nashville, Tennessee.

In May, 1943, an editorial appeared in the *Houston Post* entitled "Medical Center Takes Shape." It seemed to have been written to remind the people that the University of Texas should be complimented for being primarily responsible for the Medical Center's start. This, the editorial pointed out, was due to the foresight of the university when it located the cancer hospital and the dental school in Houston. These were busy days at the dental college as we made preparations for the opening day of the University of Texas Dental Branch.

September 1, 1943, was a new day at the dental school. It was the close of the Texas Dental College and the opening of the University of Texas Dental Branch. At eight o'clock that morning, Carroll D. Simmons, comptroller of the university, and Charles Sparenberg, his assistant, walked into my office. They introduced themselves and Simmons explained that they needed to examine all books, finances, and business operations and transfer them, as of that moment, to the University of Texas. Simmons asked me if I intended to recommend Elna Birath, who had been the business manager of the Texas Dental College, as auditor for the University of Texas Dental Branch. My reply was "yes." Sparenberg then informed me that Mrs. Birath would be the only woman in such an important position in the entire university system, intimating that a man really should fill the position. I explained to them the important role Mrs. Birath had played in keeping the Texas Dental College operating through trying times. Also, I told them that I doubted there was a man in the university system who could do better than Mrs. Birath in this capacity. I invited Mrs. Birath into my office, introduced her to the gentlemen, and explained their mission. Not too many months passed before I began to hear many favorable remarks from Mr. Simmons and Mr. Sparenberg about Mrs. Birath.

Later, in the fall of 1943, the board of regents met in Galveston. It was the first meeting of the board that I attended as an officer of the university. President Rainey had asked me to be present. Dr. Bertner was also present. At the close of the meeting Dr. Rainey asked me if I were returning to Houston. I had planned to do so, and he returned with me. During the trip back, Dr. Rainey told me of an idea he had, which he asked that I consider confidential for the time being. He informed me that he was giving considerable thought to how the university should be organized. He believed that it was now time to think about the end of the war and the need for the university to prepare for its close. In his discussion, he explained that a university could operate best if all of its schools were on one campus. "Therefore," he said, "I have decided, before it is too late, that the medical school, the dental school, and other related institutions such as the cancer hospital be located in Austin." He did not ask me to comment, so I remained silent except for one cautious remark: "Many other universities have this type of coordination." I later learned that President Rainey may have mentioned his plan to Mr. Freeman the morning after our conversation. Mr. Freeman told me years later that he thought it was about this time (1943) that President Rainey had come to his office and mentioned the matter to him, to which Freeman said he voiced strong disapproval. At the time of President Rainey's conversation with me, I decided that it would be best to wait and see if he would proceed with these plans.

During the next summer, on July 15, 1944, Dr. Rainey presented to the board of regents a printed report on "The Future Development of the University of Texas." It was an excellent and scholarly report describing a total university program. The preparation of the report reflected many hours of study, as well as a considerable amount of time that had been necessary to assemble the material, which he had used as supporting evidence. At this meeting, Dr. Rainey asked for approval of his recommendation. Without comment, the chairman of the board announced that the report would be referred to the medical committee of the board of regents. In the report, Dr. Rainey discussed at length the reasons why all units of the university should be located on the Austin campus. This, of course, included the items that he mentioned to me in our discussion. It was out in the open. He recommended that the Medical Branch, the dental branch, and the cancer hospital all be located in Austin. A vociferous and drawn out controversy developed. It became a constant pro and con debate between many different groups. It must have been that the Anderson Foundation had some indication that this might happen because of the agreement that they had made with Baylor University to bring their medical and dental schools to Houston. President Rainey's report and his strong approval of it and the equally strong disapproval of it by opposing forces (physicians and others), caused a confrontation that was a repetition of many others that had occurred between universities and practicing physicians. Yet it was my observation that where off-campus medical schools were operated by universities, they were quite successful.

Judge Dudley Woodward, Jr., chairman of the board of regents, appointed three members of the board's medical committee to serve as a special investigative committee to consider the Rainey report. Those appointed were H. H. Weinert, Orville Bullington, and Judge D. F. Strickland. The report of the committee was released in the fall of 1944. Their report recommended that Dr. Rainey's recommendation be disapproved. All schools of the university should remain in their present locations. Some time later, another special committee of seventy-five citizens confirmed their recommendations. Rex Baker, Hines Baker's brother, served as chairman of this special committee.

We were nearing the time when the medical center was to be formally organized. Dr. Bertner was busily engaged with his civil defense duties as well as with the cancer hospital. Therefore, our discussions for the organization of the medical center were not as frequent as we would have liked them to be. Mrs. Birath and I had been working during the summer and fall on the dental branch operating budget in preparation for the 1945 session of the legislature. It was necessary to have the budget request completed very early since it was to be presented first to the president and the board of regents of the university for their approval. Then it would be presented in hearings before the board of control, the governor's budget committee, and later, before the legislative budget board. Both the governor's committee and the legislative budget board presented their recommendations independently to the legislature.

We drove to Austin for each of these hearings. Prior to the presentation of the budget to the regents, meetings had been held with the faculty. All departmental requests were based upon the recommendations of the department chairman. Dr. Leake visited Houston frequently and took an active part in helping us prepare material that would be used later for appearances before various committees in Houston and throughout the state. The committees needed this information when they were discussing the legislative bills pending before the legislature.

At this time, all efforts were directed towards appropriations for buildings of the university to be located in Houston. Public appearances were made before every civic group that would invite us. In June, 1944, John Freeman gave an excellent address to the Rotary Club. He explained the aims and purposes of the medical center. This was the first address given by Freeman on behalf of the Texas Medical Center. Though not a member of Rotary at the time, Freeman had been one of its founding members. During the summer of 1944, Freeman and other members of the Anderson Foundation were discussing plans for the Medical Center's charter. He wrote a rough draft and mailed a copy of it to Dr. Bertner with a letter explaining that changes might be necessary. Dr. Bertner, in July, 1945, came by my office on his way to Hermann Hospital with a copy of the charter and a few penciled changes to it that Freeman had added. He asked that I read it. Dr. Bertner stopped by my office again on the way back to his office and said he thought it was a well-drafted instrument. Knowing little about charters, I agreed. It was not until late 1945 that the charter was presented to the secretary of state and the Texas Medical Center became a chartered, non-profit corporation. Those who signed the charter were James Anderson, Hines H. Baker, William B. Bates, E. W. Bertner, Ray L. Dudley, John H. Freeman, Clinton S. Quinn, H. M. Wilkins, and me, Frederick C. Elliott. The first meeting of the Texas Medical Center Board of Trustees was not held until December 11, 1945. Officers were elected at this meeting. The officers named were Dr. E. W. Bertner, president; Mr. John H. Freeman, vice president; Col. James Anderson, treasurer; and I was named secretary.

On Tuesday night, August 14, 1945, Ann and I had retired earlier than usual. We must have been soundly sleeping to miss the cries of the newsboys shouting, "Extry! Extry!" because it was not until early the next morning we learned by radio that the war had ended! I hurried to the dental school. No one was there but a few office personnel and the building maintenance staff. I informed the few who were there that the school would close. Every shop in the city was closed. The streets were crowded with deliriously happy people. It was the second such day in my life. I hope that I shall not see another one, even though this day was a happy one. Tears were shed for those who wouldn't be with us to participate in this joyous day. Within a short time we received information from Washington that all deferred students would be dropped back to a no-war status in the draft. The administration soon adjusted back to a peacetime schedule. We were busy preparing for a return to the four-year schedule that would begin on September 1, 1946. Now, we could move forward with a new vigor and with new enthusiasm without the anxiety of war hanging over us.

Late in the year, ground was broken for the first building to be built in the Medical Center—Baylor University College of Medicine. Hermann Hospital and its nursing school had been operating for several years on adjoining property, but not actually within the Medical Center. The groundbreaking ceremony was a happy occasion for Baylor as well as for all of us who had spent so many years working toward this day.

In December, Dr. Bertner gave the last public address of the year regarding the Medical Center. The many newspaper articles that had appeared throughout the year had prompted various citizens' groups to invite us to speak to their organizations. Citizens throughout the city were beginning to boast that Houston was to have a Medical Center second to none. It was in November that Dr. Bertner called to inform me that he had an invitation to speak at the Kiwanis Club at their first meeting in December. He asked that I get together some of the material that we had been preparing recently for the University of Texas. From this material he organized an excellent address. I was invited to the luncheon to hear Dr. Bertner speak and his address turned out to be a surprise for all us, even for Dr. Bertner, I believe. While Dr. Bertner usually followed his notes when making an address, he at times added impromptu remarks. During his address on this day, he hesitated for a moment and then said, "The Texas Medical Center within a short time will be a development that will exceed $100 million." This was a news item.

The next morning the *Houston Post* printed a full-page headline, "$100 Million Medical Center for Houston." When the news broke, Dr. Bertner was at the hospital so Colonel Bates called me and asked, "Where's Bill going to get this kind of money?" I told Colonel Bates that this was an out-of-the-blue statement made by Dr. Bertner to excite interest in the Medical Center. I am sure that the reaction was more than any of us anticipated. This headline, quoting Dr. Bertner, began to appear in newspapers throughout the United States. However, we later knew that Dr. Bertner had missed by a wide margin the actual worth the Medical Center enterprises would amass. In 1976, with buildings still under construction, the worth of the Medical Center exceeded over $400 million. Dr. Bertner's address was a happy way to end the year.

CHAPTER 4

Building a Medical Center
The First Institutions, 1946–48

THE YEARS 1944 AND 1945 passed rapidly and paved the way for a busy 1946. Many actions taken during 1946 would cause the Medical Center to move forward at a fast pace. In January, three important members joined the board of trustees: Oveta Culp Hobby, Hugh Roy Cullen, and Jesse H. Jones. It was an educational experience for me to witness the manner in which these new members quickly grasped the concept of the medical center and how they moved to determine ways for implementing the many plans that we had under consideration.[1]

Our first action for the year was one for the public—a carefully planned dinner for the dedication of the Medical Center. We considered several nationally known individuals as speakers. Finally, the speaker that I had suggested, Dr. Raymond B. Allen, president of Washington University, was chosen. I had told the trustees that Dr. Allen, just prior to his appointment as president of Washington University, had been executive dean of the University of Illinois College of Medicine and director of the Chicago campus of the university, which consisted entirely of medical and dental institutions. He served also as the chief development officer of the Chicago Medical Center, one of the first medical centers in the United States to be designated by this title. The Chicago Medical Center consisted of many other institutions that were operated by others; all were engaged in medical and dental education. Also, several different types of hospitals and other institutions were located in the same neighborhood. Dr. Allen's particular assignment was to bring these institutions, which were operated by different groups and administered by several different administrators, into a cooperative endeavor. This was a difficult task and we were to learn later how difficult it really was.

On February 28, 1946, the dedication was held in the Rice Hotel, then the home of John Freeman, Dr. Bertner, and Jesse Jones. The Rice Hotel's large banquet room was filled to capacity. Over six hundred citizens of Houston showed that they were behind the Texas Medical Center. It was a proud moment for Col. George A. Hill, Jr., who had given so much of his

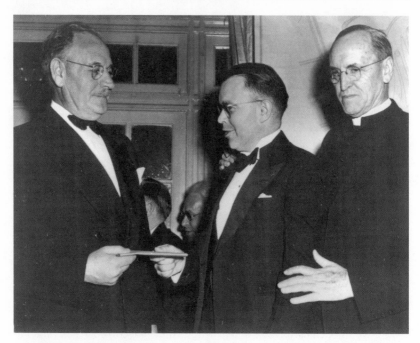

W. Leland Anderson presents the deed for the original 134 acres of land to
Dr. Ernst W. Bertner at the dedicatory dinner for Texas Medical Center,
February 28, 1946. From left: Dr. E. W. Bertner, W. Leland Anderson, and
Episcopal Bishop Clinton S. Quinn. Courtesy Mavis P. Kelsey, Sr.

time to Texas Medical Center projects. He could take pride in the remarks that he made since he was largely responsible for what had happened. He said, "At this time the projects which have been approved for inclusion in the Texas Medical Center by the trustees, or the regents of the university or the governing bodies concerned therewith are as follows: first, Baylor University Medical School; second, University of Houston nursing program; third, Rice Institute Cooperative Program for Research; fourth, nine projects of the University of Texas as follows." Then he named the projects of the university: the M. D. Anderson Hospital for Cancer Research; the School of Medicine preceptor training program; the postgraduate and graduate Schools of Medicine; the School of Dentistry; the College of Dental Nursing; the postgraduate and graduate Schools of Dentistry; the Institute of Orthodontics; the School of Public Health; and, the Institute of Geographic Medicine. He had omitted one—the Institute of Gerontology. He also mentioned five hospitals: Hermann Hospital, St. Luke's Hospital, Methodist Hospital, the tuberculosis hospital, and Shrine Children's Hospital. He continued by saying that the Houston Academy of Medicine library also was to be located in the Medical Center and a United States naval hospital was to be constructed. This later became the United States Veterans Administration Hospital. Following Hill's address, Dr. Allen explained to the board and to all of the citizens how fortunate they were to have such a plan under development.[2]

The ideas and plans for so many of the institutions that Colonel Hill named were being studied for quite some time before his announcement was made. The information that had been gathered together was later used in preparing plans that were drafted for the Medical Center institutions. During the year preceding the dedication exercises, Dr. Bertner, Dr. Leake, myself, and a large number of others had worked on the development of the plans. During the fall of 1945, we had completed our plans to the degree that H. A. Kipp could include them in his final study for that year. "Plan Number 20-A," prepared by Kipp, was printed in December, 1945. On this plat plan, Kipp indicated the locations of the institutions and gave each one of them a number. In addition to those that Colonel Hill had mentioned in his dedicatory address, Kipp included Hermann Hospital, Hermann Hospital School of Nursing, the Hermann intern home, and a Hermann outpatient clinic. Also included were the Children's Hospital, the urological hospital, the Hermann professional building, the convalescent hospital, and the U.S. Marine hospital.

Several facilities were included that the Medical Center would operate, including the central power plant, the animal house, the laundry, the greenhouse, and the maintenance building. These facilities would serve all of the institutions in the Medical Center. Finally, Kipp had included sites for apartments and smaller lots for the construction of doctors' homes. How little did we realize at the time that what we thought was to be an overabundance of land was later to be so inadequate, even for the educational and research institutions that were to come. Certainly there was no room for doctors' homes and resident apartments. Several of the institutions named were never developed. However, many that were not mentioned have taken their place.

In late 1945, I began to work with Hulon Black, director of development for the University of Texas, on the development of plans for the promotion of the university in the Texas Medical Center. The relationship of the development board to the board of regents was one that I later, in 1962, patterned a plan after. The University of Texas development board was organized in 1938 for the purpose of interesting private philanthropy in projects for which appropriations from the legislature would be difficult to obtain. The first officers of the development board were Hines H. Baker, president of Humble Oil and Refining Company (later to become Exxon), Col. George Hill, president of the Houston Oil Company, and J. R. Parten, president of Woodley Petroleum Company. Other members of the board were appointed from the faculty. The board and the director for development reported to the board of regents. The plan I recommended followed this procedure with the exception that the development committee of the Texas Medical Center's board of trustees would comprise members of the board.[3]

We were collaborating on the preparation of a brochure that would serve as material to present the aims and purposes of the university programs in the Texas Medical Center. Dr. Bertner assisted us as much as possible, but his days were more than overfilled. Chauncey Leake, vice president for medical affairs, was also of great help. At a dinner given for Dr. Leake by the chamber of commerce, he mentioned several other institutions that he had discussed with us, which he believed should be included in the University of Texas program in Houston. These were approved by the board of regents, after which they were included in the previously mentioned groups. Hulon Black wanted pictures of the two buildings that had been approved for immediate construction included in the brochure. It was not easy to get illustrations for buildings not yet planned, and it created somewhat of a problem since time was short. Hulon Black suggested that Leon White, the architect for the university who had planned several campus buildings, be asked to picture buildings that he thought might serve the purpose. White imagined what a dental school and cancer hospital might look like after Dr. Leake, Dr. Bertner, and I had discussed them with him. His imagination was excellent and we used the pictures he created in the brochure, "The University of Texas in the Texas Medical Center," which the development board published in early 1946. Hulon Black had done an excellent job of rewriting the material that we had prepared for him. The brochure included illustrations of the buildings, as well as reproductions of letters from the chairman of the board of regents, officers of state and local medical and dental associations, and one from Dr. Bertner as president of the Medical Center.

The publication created considerable interest. It was widely distributed in Houston and throughout the state. Also, we were pressed for time in the production of the brochure since the officers of the Texas Exes wanted to distribute it to those attending a take-off dinner in Houston on March 3, 1946.

Again, the Rice Hotel's ballroom was filled to capacity. The newspapers carried excellent front page stories about the discussions and the announcements made by the chairman of the board of regents. They were illustrated with many pictures, including White's renditions of the Dental Branch building and the cancer hospital. Black and I were pleased with the quotes that appeared in the newspapers that had been lifted from our brochure. The special fund drive committee of the chamber of commerce had been appointed and a "Committee of 100" of the Texas Exes was assigned to assist them. It was only a short time later on April 17, 1946, that the newspaper headlines announced: "First Funds Given to Committee."

It seemed that all the pent-up energies for good that had been submerged because of the war were now being released in full force. Everyone was working. Those of us in the Medical Center—Dr. Bertner and institutional heads—were extremely interested and assisted the committee when asked to do so. Our chief interest was the planning of the multiple activities that were underway. It was necessary that frequent Medical Center board conferences were held with different individuals and groups. Agreements had to be reached with the two gas companies and with the light and telephone companies concerning utility lines to be laid underground in the Medical Center. Also, we held conferences with city officials, the University of Texas, and with Baylor University College of Medicine officials. The faculty of the Dental Branch was planning space for their departments in the new branch building. The architects needed their plans. It seemed that almost every architect in Houston was involved in developing plans for Medical Center buildings. On March 28, 1946, President Truman signed a bill creating a veterans hospital for Houston. Later this was associated with the teaching programs at Baylor University College of Medicine and the University of Texas Dental Branch. A surprise gift was given to the Medical Center by Mr. and Mrs. Norman Purchase—a building for the cancer hospital.

The future of the Medical Center began to emerge in 1946. Events occurred during this year that would guide the growth and destiny of the Medical Center for some time to come. Naturally, it was a year of firsts since it was the first year after its organization. Early in April, the dynamic Warren Bellows, Sr., was appointed chairman of the chamber of commerce's large "Committee of 75." He brought the fund drive, which had been languishing, to a successful conclusion. He became quite interested in the Medical Center and its projects. Later he served as a member of the Anderson Foundation Board of Trustees and a member of the Cancer Foundation Board of Visitors.

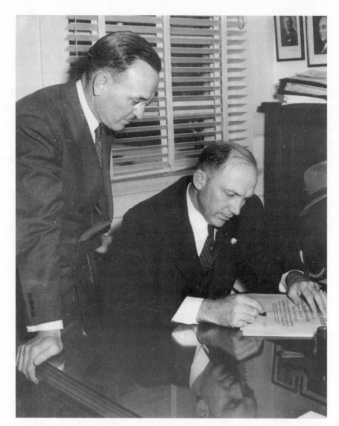

Elliott with Dr. Homer P. Rainey, signing diplomas, circa 1944.
Courtesy E. W. D'Anton

In May, a picture of the library for the Medical Center was printed in the *Houston Post*. Dr. Moise Levy, president of the Houston Academy of Medicine, announced that the estimated cost of the building was $565,000, for which the Anderson Foundation and Jesse Jones had provided the funds. In addition to the library, the building would provide offices for several medical organizations, including the Texas Medical Center and the Harris County Medical Society.

J. W. Neal, wife of the founder of the Maxwell House coffee company, gave another sizeable gift of twenty-five thousand dollars to the chamber of commerce committee for the M. D. Anderson Hospital.[4] This gift was followed by hundreds of other gifts, large and small. One of the lesser events for the year, as announced in the newspaper in July, was "Dr. Frederick C.

Elliott was named as vice president of the University of Texas, as well as dean of the dental branch in Houston." "In effect," the article stated, "creation of the new job raised the hitherto small dental school to a status equal to that of the University of Texas Medical Branch in Galveston, headed by Dr. Chauncey Leake." Early in July, William A. Kirkland, executive vice president of the First National Bank, became a member of the Texas Medical Center Board of Trustees. Many times his banking experience served the board of trustees well when they needed sound financial advice. He had helped also, to a large degree, in the development of Rice Institute and was a member of their board.[5]

On a Saturday in July, 1946, I was introduced to a lieutenant colonel in the air force—R. Lee Clark. Those of us in the office of the University of Texas president who were introduced to Dr. Clark were Dr. E. W. Bertner, Dr. Chauncey Leake, and Dr. Wilson H. Elkins, president of Texas Western College in El Paso, which was a responsibility of the University of Texas Board of Regents. Dr. Theophilus S. Painter, acting president of the university, had asked Lieutenant Colonel Clark to be present at this meeting of the board of regents. Dr. Bertner and Dr. Painter had met with him previously. They were convinced that he was the man that they wanted to recommend to the board of regents to become the first director of the M. D. Anderson Hospital for Cancer Research in Houston. All of us present took a liking to Dr. Clark. He was a pleasant, soft spoken, attentive young man. He was ushered into the meeting of the board of regents, and it was not long until we were invited into the board meeting to meet the new director of the M. D. Anderson Hospital.

The next week Dr. Clark visited Houston. He was quite pleased with the accomplishments Dr. Bertner had made in such a short time and was of the opinion that the Texas Medical Center had a great future. In a conversation with a reporter he remarked, "Houston is a city that will make Texas brags come true. The cancer hospital will become a world center in the field of cancer research." He mentioned, too, that "there is a possibility that another field in cancer research would be developed—that of radioactivity." He related this assertion to the effects of the atomic bomb. We soon were to learn that Dr. Clark was a man of vision. Very early, after Dr. Clark arrived in Houston, he changed the name and title of the hospital because he felt that the word "research" did not express the true purposes for which the hospital was to be developed. In his opinion, it was to be for patients. Research would be done elsewhere, in quarters that were equipped for this purpose. It was not long until his wife, also a physician, and his two children, a nine-year-old girl and a seven-year-old boy, arrived in Houston. The association that I developed with Dr. Clark became one of the real happenings in my life.[6]

Stories about the Medical Center and its development appeared almost daily in all of the Houston newspapers. Each story was illustrated with either architects' renditions or actual photographs of buildings under construction.[7] The Hermann Professional Building was announced and pictured as part of the Medical Center. It was not on Medical Center property, but it was to provide office space for physicians who were connected with the hospitals or schools in the Medical Center. Also, in the same article, another picture appeared of the new building for Hermann Hospital. The new Hermann Hospital adjoined the old building, which had been in operation for some time. It too was to serve physicians, both from the schools of the Medical Center and those who had offices in the Hermann Professional Building.[8] Later, another story and picture appeared about the new Methodist Hospital that was to be constructed in the Medical Center. This was history for Methodist Hospital and a proud day for Josie Roberts, the administrator. She had worked for many years for a new hospital. Her years of administration had proved successful in the old hospital located on San Jacinto Street. Many of Houston's most prominent physicians were on the Methodist staff at the old location. Many of them continued to serve in their various specialties in the new hospital.[9]

The Texas Medical Center trustees then decided that we should have professional consultants study the Medical Center plans. We were not in a position to estimate the number of hospital beds that might be required for the center in the future. James A. Hamilton and Associates of New Haven, Connecticut, were retained for this purpose. It was necessary that the study be made not only for the Medical Center, but that it must include the needs of all the facilities such as hospitals, clinics, and others that were located in the greater Houston area and Harris County. When Hamilton gave the report of his studies to the board of trustees, we learned that we had not over planned as some members of the board had thought, but rather that our plans were not extensive enough.[10]

The Medical Center was making real news. Many stories appeared in newspapers and magazines throughout Texas and the United States. These stories were nice to read, yet they caused a little doubt to creep into our minds as to whether we could live up to it all. A quote from the *Washington Sun* on August 27, 1946, explains why we had this doubt in our minds: "Some government medical authorities believe that Houston, Texas is by way of becoming the Medical Center of both North and South America.

Houston's $100 million Medical Center program got underway with scant notice, but other cities are perking up at its immensity." Continuing, the article stated, "Medics think the Houston plan for its center, on a 161 acre plot, is the best thought out in America." The 161 acres mentioned in the article, no doubt, also included the land that was given to the government by citizens of Houston for the construction of the veterans hospital. The veterans hospital was considered a part of the Texas Medical Center.

Dr. Bertner approached Sue Barnett, an outstanding newspaper reporter who had previously served for some time with the Houston Planning Commission, and asked her to serve with him as his assistant in promoting the Medical Center. The widespread public recognition of the Medical Center was largely due to Barnett's journalistic ability. Dr. Bertner had asked her to serve for a short time on a temporary basis, but her short time stretched from almost the beginning of the Medical Center until her retirement in 1953. She played an important part in helping to organize the various functions of the Medical Center working with Dr. Bertner full-time as his administrative assistant. Mrs. Barnett and I also worked closely together throughout the early years. We prepared many articles together. She recorded the minutes of the board of trustees and the executive committee meetings, which relieved me of the responsibility. While Sue Barnett could not recall her visits with me in Memphis, she had called upon me at the University of Tennessee Dental School when I was on the faculty there. She was the medical reporter for the leading newspaper of Tennessee, the *Memphis Commercial Appeal.* She authored Medical Center brochures and she published a monthly newspaper, *The Texas Medical Center News,* that many people throughout the United States read with interest. It was discontinued when she retired from the Medical Center.

While I will not discuss the Medical Center's board of trustee meetings in detail, there are some events that were significant as far as the development of the center was concerned that occurred during 1946. At the July meeting, the trustees decided that an executive committee should be authorized. The executive committee would meet frequently and dispense with the day-by-day items that required approval. These actions would be reported later to the board of trustees for ratification. Colonel James Anderson, the treasurer of the board, recommended that an assistant treasurer should be appointed. His recommendation was approved and an assistant treasurer, J. M. Jackson, was appointed in September. James A. Hamilton had made a cursory report to the board of trustees earlier in the year. In October, Hamilton had completed his studies and reported in detail. Some of his predictions were interesting and many of his recommendations were of utmost importance. He said that in 1970, Houston would have a population of 1,474,415. In 1970, the U. S. census reported that the actual population of Houston was 1,232,800, and that the population of greater Houston was 1,741,912. Hamilton also had estimated the number of hospital beds that would be needed. His estimates, in all categories were quite extensive. He stated that a two hundred-bed hospital would be needed for acute illnesses and three thousand beds would be needed for the Medical Center. In addition, he gave figures for each category of beds needed: five hundred for chronic diseases, seven hundred for children's diseases, and three hundred psychiatric beds. He also said that an outpatient clinic, including a central pathologic unit, a central emergency and receiving unit, a central ambulance service, and a central medical records service was critical for the Medical Center. He also recommended that a central maintenance department be established, along with a central linen and laundry facility, a central manufacturing pharmacy, a central blood bank, and a central personnel department. We had actually mentioned some of these before the Hamilton report. He recommended that by 1952, the Medical Center should have a central school of nursing to graduate three hundred nurses a year and that we should have a college of nursing that would accommodate nine hundred students on a four-year term basis. He made other organizational recommendations.

We were pleased with Hamilton's report; it was thorough and well done, and he gave valid reasons for each of his recommendations. Viewing the Medical Center today, some of his recommendations may be observed operation, but most of his recommendations for central operations were not carried out. Dr. Bertner and I moved forward, though, to bring many of his recommendations into reality. We, and other members of the Medical Center's board, were to be disappointed. There was criticism of one of the central facilities that had been recommended that resulted in a long, continuing resistance to many of the other hoped-for cooperative operations. I believe that if Hamilton's recommendations had been carried out and put into operation, that the facilities provided would have been most beneficial to all institutions in the Medical Center.

Dr. R. Lee Clark was present at a meeting of the Texas Medical Center Board of Trustees on November 26, 1946. He was invited so that the trustees could meet the new director of the M. D. Anderson Hospital for Cancer Research. Dr. Clark reported the activities that he had completed since his arrival. Hines Baker, in complimenting Dr. Clark, also suggested, "that the cancer hospital not get too involved in organizational work and neglect its true function of research." Baker would later know that he need not have had any doubts. Colonel Bates and Dr. Bertner both invited Dr. Clark to attend all future meetings of the Medical Center trustees, which was heartily agreed to by all the trustees present. Dr. Clark appreciated the invitation, however, he never attended a meeting of the Texas Medical Center board unless he could bring the board information that he felt would be of interest and benefit to them.

It was in the latter part of December that the plan for the Children's Hospital was announced. Dr. David Greer was largely responsible for the enthusiastic support of this project by the Houston Pediatric Society. All through 1946, a whirlwind of announcements was made about various projects that were desired within the Medical Center. All of these announcements caused a continued flurry of excitement in the minds of citizens of Houston from every walk of life. Yet funds were needed if these dreams of the people were to become a reality.

The days were too short for Dr. Clark and me. Our daily administrative activities required constant attention. Yet, we found time to dream and plan for other institutions for the Medical Center. We made frequent trips to Austin to discuss with the university officials our budgets and the supporting material we were preparing for the legislature. This was a new experience for us both. Dr. Clark and I would ask for funds, not only for our operating budget, but also for the construction of the buildings, both for the cancer hospital and for the dental branch. Much to our surprise, we learned that this could not be done until the board of regents had obtained legislative approval to locate the university buildings in the Texas Medical Center. When this matter came before the legislature, Dr. Clark and I were surprised at the objections raised by some of the legislators to locating university buildings in the Texas Medical Center. However, their objections were out-voted and approval was granted to the board of regents for the Houston project.

For Dr. Clark and for me, the many trips we made to Austin were pleasurable. Lee and I were together constantly, and our conversations were filled with dreams and plans. We were both avid listeners and tried out our new ideas on each other. He would add building blocks to my dreams and I would add to his. Throughout all of our discussions, we had one common thought: that whatever developed from our dreams must result in building a better health future for all. Our chief concern was prevention, even though we knew our plans for treatment had to be pursued, crystallized, and taught better in our institution than anywhere else in the world. What visions of hope we both held! We learned through the years that divine guidance was our real hope. We did not approach our many appearances before legislative committees or our conversations with individual legislators and others with any thought of failure because we were not "alone" in our efforts.

We were pleased when the Texas Exes "Committee of 100" and the chamber of commerce invited the legislature, as a body, to visit Houston and learn firsthand what the Texas Medical Center had to offer to the people of Texas. Colonel George Hill, the chairman of the development board of the University of Texas, had invited the board of regents to Houston before the announcement of the visit of the legislators was made. He wanted to ascertain from the regents what might be said to the legislators when they visited Houston. This was a wise decision on Hill's part. It was at this meeting of the regents that they decided to request an appropriation of two million dollars from the legislators for the Houston project of the University of Texas. Following the meeting, Chairman Dudley Woodward remarked to a reporter, "I have no doubt that they (the legislators) will subscribe funds for the four schools of the university after seeing the project." President Painter added, "Facilities for research will be second to none in the world." In his remarks to the reporters, Colonel Hill said, "I consider this a very historic occasion. I think the matters taking place here are of transcending importance." Lee and I were not alone.

The legislature accepted the invitation and came to Houston on a special Southern Pacific Railroad train. We were all there to greet them. It was a busy day. Special buses had been provided for them to reach the various activities that had been planned. While they were highly entertained, the Medical Center was the principal objective of their visit. Lee and I were now sure that the appropriations for our buildings were in the bag. We did not hear of anything that made us think the bill would not pass. We soon learned, much to our sorrow, that our bag had a hole in it. The legislature granted approval for the university to operate in the Texas Medical Center, but no appropriations were made. This portion of the bill had been removed from the measure that passed.[11]

During the time that we devoted to the legislature, other projects for the Medical Center had not stood still. St. Luke's started a drive for one million dollars for their hospital. Likewise, Methodist Hospital started their drive. Both of these drives were announced on January 19, 1947. It was also announced early in 1947 that on December 2, 1946, the regents of the University of Texas had allocated $315,080 of the Rosalie B. Hite assets to the foundation for the building of the M. D. Anderson Cancer Hospital. Also, in early December, two financial bombshells hit Houston with a delightful and astonishing bang, just fifteen days apart. A report from California appeared

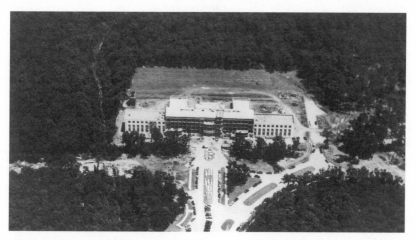

Baylor College of Medicine's Cullen Building, 1946. Courtesy Texas Medical Center

in the newspaper stating that Howard Hughes was creating a foundation for medical science with headquarters in Houston. The assets of the foundation would be $125 million. This bomb, however, failed to explode. The other was an announcement that Mr. and Mrs. Roy Cullen had established the Cullen Foundation. Roy Cullen estimated that the worth of the foundation would be approximately $80 million. This amount, Cullen thought, might later double. The Cullens were to become the benefactors to untold thousands of people in the future.[12]

The officers and trustees of the Medical Center were pleased with the enthusiastic way the growing Medical Center was being received. At our first meeting on January 14, 1947, the board passed a resolution expressing our appreciation to the many donors who had made gifts to the Medical Center institutions during the year, totaling more than $500,000. These were not gifts from large foundations, but sizable gifts from ten individual donors. On March 10, 1947, another article appeared concerning Howard Hughes and his millions. When interviewed by a reporter, Dr. Bertner said, "Public announcement of Hughes' great gift is a source of deep gratification to the Medical Center board." Yet quietly, Dr. Bertner and I thought it best that we not count our chickens until they were hatched. Articles continued to appear from time to time about Hughes, his money, and the foundation. Howard Hughes personally had withdrawn from the limelight, though, because of the many stories that were surfacing about him and his manner of living.[13]

In March, 1947, we had first learned about the new Cullen Foundation, but it was not until later that we read about Mr. and Mrs. Cullen giving three large gifts to Medical Center institutions. These gifts created widespread praise for the Cullens. Gifts of one million dollars each were given to Methodist Hospital, to Baptist Memorial Hospital, and to St. Luke's Hospital. Other gifts were given to Baylor Medical College and to Hermann Hospital. The Cullens had also given four million dollars to the University of Houston though the years. The first gift that they gave to the University of Houston was a building. It was named the Roy G. Cullen Building for their son who had been killed in an oil-field accident while working, as his father had done, on an oil rig. When the announcement was made about the formation of the foundation, the Cullen's daughters—Mrs. Lillie Cranz Portanova, Mrs. Isaac Arnold, Mrs. Douglas B. Marshall, and Mrs. Corbin Robertson—all wished to remain silently in the background. They quietly shared in praising their parents along with the public. At the trustees meeting in April, 1947, a resolution was passed that expressed the trustee's sincere appreciation of Mr. and Mrs. Roy Cullen. I have many pleasant memories of the moments I spent with Roy Cullen discussing affairs of the Medical Center as well as listening to his conversations about other matters. I admired him greatly for his vision and his fearless, forthright manner in expressing his honest concern over the welfare of our nation. He did not hesitate to call a spade a spade. As he saw it, Russia was a great menace to our nation. He felt Washington was "something else." He said to me, "If Washington does not stop giving everything away, we will have a great calamity happen to our nation." I remember one day I remarked to him that on each of my trips to Austin I thought of him as I passed by his country place. I have never forgotten his reply to me. "You know, Elliott," he said, "I like to go up there for the weekend, just Lillie and I. She cooks the meals and I help her with the dishes. Just like many of our old times together." What a fine person to have known.[14]

At the same April meeting that we passed the Cullen resolution, Dr. Bertner reported on his meeting with the administrators of all institutions in the Medical Center concerning a central heating and cooling plant. They agreed with the idea. He stated that the estimated cost of this facility was $1.85 million. This matter was referred to Leland Anderson, vice president of the board, for further study. On May 27, 1947, Anderson reported to the trustees that from information that he had obtained, he would recommend that the plan be deferred until the plan's use would justify its cost and the cost of operation.

In a memorandum that I mailed to the board of trustees, I recommended that a central plan for television installation should be developed for teaching purposes and for the interchange of conferences between institutions in the Medical Center. I reported that it was imperative that this be done as soon as possible so that it could be included by the architects in the current plans they were developing for the buildings that they were designing at the time. The required chases for the television cable could be included inexpensively at this time. Later, it would be an expensive procedure. Chases for television had been provided in the plan for the M. D. Anderson Hospital and for the Dental Branch at very little cost.

At one of our meetings of the board of trustees, we discussed how we might develop a closer working relationship between each institution. There was no doubt that many of the services requiring extensive equipment could be done in one hospital since it would be an expensive procedure for each institution to individually provide the essential equipment. Likewise, it would be costly for each institution to employ the specially trained professionals that would be needed to operate the equipment. Our discussion centered around such equipment as the artificial kidney, the cobalt unit, and other radiation therapy equipment, as well as other types of equipment. These items were indeed costly. We believed that the institutions should consider this idea before it was too late. Dr. Bertner requested that I bring a plan for institutional coordination to the board. At the meeting on June 26, 1947, I recommended that the Medical Center's board of trustees appoint a coordinating council. The administrative officer of each institution was to serve as a member of the council. The plan was approved and the council of administrators was appointed. Many of the future actions taken by the board of trustees were based upon the recommendations of the council. Also, at some meetings, questions were asked about how the Medical Center could become actively engaged in administering many of the functions of the institutions that were common to all. This question pertained primarily to patient care. Now it seemed that we were back to the problems of institutional cooperation. Yet, as these questions were studied, it became clear that it was necessary to give thought on how the educational programs of the institutions would be coordinated so that students could understand and appreciate the interrelationships of the services other professionals were to provide. By this method of teaching, each graduate would become informed as to when to consult and when to refer.

During this time, John Freeman and Dr. Bertner were visiting other medical centers in the United States where coordinated programs were underway. One in the east, Baker Memorial Pavilion of Massachusetts General Hospital in Boston, had impressed Freeman. Dr. Bertner discussed his many visits to the Mayo Clinic in Rochester. He liked their plan of coordination. I, too, had expressed to the board my understanding of the Mayo Clinic plan because they included a dental clinic in their operations. I pointed out that these operations served to bring all medical and dental disciplines together. Also, I mentioned that at the time, the graduate school of the University of Minnesota was associated with the Mayo Clinic. The board of trustees asked Dr. Bertner and I to develop a similar plan for their consideration. Dr. Bertner and I decided that whatever we developed would need to be operated by the Medical Center, but that it should be staffed by a joint endeavor of all the institutions in the center. I mailed an outline of the plan to the members of the board. The board of trustees met on July 28, 1947. James Anderson, who had been asked to serve as chairman of the newly formed clinic committee of the trustees, during the discussion of this proposed plan stated, "The Medical Center should control and operate the central out-patient clinic." He also said that if this is not done, "we will have ten or fifteen entities each governed by independent boards." The plan for the clinic was approved with recommendations that further study be given to it. James Hamilton had earlier recommended such a plan in his report.

An interesting note was added to the transactions of the trustees meeting in October when Dr. Bertner remarked, "The University of Texas Public Health School can be started soon if an additional grant of $500,000 can be obtained from the federal government." A previous grant had been allocated to the city-county plan for health centers. Neither of these grants was made because no matching funds were made available. Dr. Bertner added, "If these funds were made available the Marine Hospital would also become a reality in the Medical Center." A tract of ground already had been reserved for this purpose.

Dr. Bertner, in reporting to the board of trustees the accomplishments that had been completed in the Medical Center for the year 1947, also included his recommendations for 1948. At the top of his list of recommendations was that "an all out concerted effort should be made for an endowment for the operation of the Medical Center." Second, he recommended that the outpatient plan be carried forward. Third, he asked the trustees "to support the efforts of the Health Committee of the Chamber of Commerce, of which Dr. Elliott is chairman, in their attempt to bring about a consolidation of the city and county health departments." Later the city and county officials did agree for the county to operate the Jefferson Davis Hospital, but the health departments still remained separate. Dr. Bertner then reported that plans had been completed for the operation of the University of Houston School of Nursing in the Medical Center. Hospital training was to be given in Hermann Hospital, and the basic science courses were to be taught at the university.

Many discussions were held during the latter part of 1947 concerning the serious situation that confronted the Medical Center due to the lack of flood control for Braes Bayou. Many of the members of the Medical Center board had attended meetings of the city council at the time that the flood control program was considered. On January 19, 1948, a large group of Houston citizens, headed by Dr. Bertner, appeared before the Army Corps of Engineers in Washington. The group included Mayor Oscar Holcombe and County Judge Glenn Perry. Also among the group were representatives from many of the institutions in the Medical Center and other institutions nearby. Those represented were the Rice Institute, the Shamrock Hotel, and the navy hospital. I represented several others. Those of us from the Medical Center flew to Washington in the private plane of George and Herman Brown. This was a successful venture since the flood control program was approved. Flooding of much of this section of Houston had occurred in 1929 and 1935. At one time Baylor had built dikes around their building to prevent flooding of the ground floor, but it still was flooded before the Braes Bayou work had been completed.[15]

Plans were moving forward for the many buildings that were to be located in the Medical Center. Several tracts of land had not yet been deeded. At a trustee meeting held to consider these deeds, Colonel Bates presented a resolution that would change the deed restrictions. It would require the institutions to cooperate with the plan for the outpatient clinic in the Medical Center. At the meeting, it was decided to allocate the tracts of ground to the several institutions. However, their deeds would not be completed until the restrictions concerning the outpatient clinic had been included in them. Once this action was completed, they would receive deeds to their land. The land tracts granted at this meeting were to Methodist Hospital, Children's Hospital, St. Luke's Hospital, and to the University of Texas. Later it became necessary to remove the restrictions contained in the University of Texas deed since the attorney general would not accept a deed of property to the state of Texas that included any type of restriction. The restrictions that were deleted from the deeds were included in a special instrument, which was approved by the board of regents as a part of their agreement. No disagreements with the University of Texas have resulted because of this omission. Also, at this meeting Dr. Bertner reported that he had received a request for land from the officers of the Young Men's Christian Association (YMCA). After some discussion, Dr. Bertner was requested to inform the YMCA officers that while it was an excellent idea to have a YMCA near the Medical Center, it could not be located in the Medical Center. By charter, institutions in the Medical Center must be medical institutions.[16]

On April 24, 1948, Baylor dedicated their new medical college building. This was a highlight of the year since it was the first building to be completed in the Medical Center. The dedication was a three day affair. Several notable visitors took part in the program, including Secretary of the Army Kenneth C. Royall; Dr. William R. White, president of Baylor University; Dr. B. Harvie Branscomb, chancellor of Vanderbilt University; and many other important guests. There were over five hundred friends of Baylor present for the dedication of the Cullen building. Funds for the building had been given by Mr. and Mrs. Roy Cullen and by the Anderson Foundation, the Cullens giving $800,000 and the Anderson Foundation providing $1 million dollars. The Anderson Foundation also had given $1 million over a ten year period for operating expenses. Ray L. Dudley, a trustee of both Baylor Medical College and the Medical Center, was presiding at the ceremonies when portraits of Roy and Lillie Cullen and Monroe D. Anderson were unveiled. "These portraits," said Dudley, "shall hang in the auditorium as long as there is a Baylor."[17]

Once again, at the trustee meeting of the Medical Center on June 21, the outpatient clinic and pathologic institute were discussed. At the close of the discussion, Roy Cullen remarked that he would ask the trustees of the Cullen Foundation to pay for the total cost of the outpatient clinic, but he asked that the decision presently be kept confidential. Further, Cullen said, "For the development of this great Medical Center, we must have a tie-rod and this institution is it." He continued, "We can't start the Medical Center without it . . . there are no selfish purposes in the membership of this board. There are no political ambitions or any financial gains to be made. This board here must be the final authority in every case of policy making." In an expression of appreciation to Cullen for this generous offer, I said, "As the only representative present of an institution operating in the Medical Center, I want to thank you, Mr. Cullen, for this generous offer, since when the out-patient clinic is completed, the dental school will have a far greater opportunity for development than it would have had."

At their meeting on July 26, the city council approved a resolution authorizing the mayor to ask for a federal grant of $500,000 that the city wished to use to match $1.8 million of unissued bonds for the construction of a tuberculosis hospital in the Medical Center. Ground had been reserved for some time for this hospital. All of the institutions in the Medical Center were moving forward with their programs.[18]

Baylor was making rapid progress in the development of their departments and in the procurement of outstanding members for their faculty. Several positions on the faculty were open since many of the former faculty members remained in Dallas at the time that Baylor Medical School moved to Houston. Baylor announced in August that Dr. Michael DeBakey had been appointed the new professor of surgery. He had been associate professor of surgery at Tulane University School of Medicine in New Orleans, Louisiana. Dr. DeBakey was appointed the Judson L. Taylor Professor of Surgery and chairman of the department. The department was named after Dr. Taylor because of his outstanding service to the medical profession. Dr. Taylor had served as a professor of surgery until the time of his death. A native of Lake Charles, Louisiana, he had been a prominent member of the board of trustees of the Texas Dental College, as well as a professor of surgery prior to his appointment as a member of the board of regents of the University of Texas. He received his bachelor of science degree from Tulane University in 1930 and his medical doctor degree from the same university in 1932. In 1935, he received a master of science degree in surgery from Tulane. His accomplishments throughout the years were noted many times in newspapers and publications throughout the world. Dr. DeBakey was a leading research surgeon in the United States. His development of artificial materials for replacement of diseased arteries was a notable contribution to surgery. In the beginning, he did all of his own sewing of the artificial material that he used in surgery. Later, manufacturers loomed the material into the many different sizes that he needed. Dr. DeBakey and Dr. Denton Cooley, through the years, became a well-known team in the field of arteriole-vascular surgery and open-heart surgery. Dr. Denton Cooley was the son of Dr. Ralph Cooley, Sr., a member of the board of trustees and a faculty member of the dental college for quite some time. Drs. DeBakey and Cooley became widely known at the time that they began transplanting human hearts. It is this fearless approach to such conditions that is a necessary part of medical research.[19]

In September, Dr. R. Lee Clark was appointed dean of the Baylor's Postgraduate School of Medicine. Dr. Clark accepted this appointment so that the school could begin operations immediately. The school opened in the temporary quarters of the M. D. Anderson Hospital for Cancer Research. Six students were enrolled as graduate students the first year. The faculty consisted of faculty members of the Medical Branch of Galveston, the M. D. Anderson Hospital, and the Dental Branch.

It had been a busy year for those of us who were putting the Medical Center together and doubly so for the teams of the cancer hospital and the Dental Branch. In addition, the Medical Center duties were increasing. Time had to be set aside to prepare for the upcoming session of the legislature, not only for the operating budget of the Houston branch of the University of Texas, but also because we were to renew our requests for building funds. Our team at the Dental Branch held session after session at night with our architects to develop and finalize plans for our hoped-for new building. The completed plans were indeed an innovative accomplishment of our team and of our architects, Fred MacKie and Karl Kamrath. A new concept of teaching had been developed, and an entirely new design for a dental school building had been created.

Likewise, the same efforts had been underway by Dr. Clark and his team. His dream was an entirely new concept in hospital design and function to coordinate the research laboratories, the diagnostic clinic, and the patient care facilities. Dr. Clark, in order to be in a position to explain his plans to the architects, spent many hours studying architecture. The Dental Branch and the cancer hospital plans were to be given widespread coverage by newspapers and magazines throughout the United States. The Georgia pink marble exterior planned for both buildings captured the eye of all of those who admired beauty. When Lee and I saw the architects' renditions of the buildings for the first time, had one closely observing, they might have seen a glisten in our eyes. It was Lee who discovered the Georgia pink marble and had convinced the architects that it would be practical to use the marble for the exteriors of both buildings. Along with the construction engineers, the architects had to develop a new type of construction so that as little of the marble as possible would be used. It was not available in quantities sufficient for large, block-type construction. Slabs of about one-and-a-half to two inches thick were cut and used as an "exterior skin." The Houston building code had to be changed by the city council so that this type of construction would be allowed in the city's building code. Now, with beautiful renditions of these buildings and with explicitly detailed notes, Lee and I were ready for the beginning of 1949, when the next legislative session would convene.

CHAPTER 5

Working Together
Public Funds and Private Philanthropy

BY JANUARY, 1949, THE OFFICE STAFF of the Dental Branch had assembled a large amount of information concerning the need for a new building. They prepared some of the material for the legislators and developed
other packets for distribution to our many supporters throughout the state.
It was necessary that we not allow our friends to relax their efforts since the
Dental Branch was now a university school. We had to remind them that we
still needed funds for a building in which the school could operate. One of
our enthusiastic supporters, Al Collins, wrote an article that appeared in the
Houston Chronicle on January 17, 1949. The half-page article appealed for
support of our $2.5 million request from the legislature for the construction
of the building. The estimated cost of the building was $4.25 million. A
grant from the M. D. Anderson Foundation and funds from other sources
would be matched with the state appropriations. Collins based his story on
material provided by the office staff of the Dental College. He wrote the
story as if the statements made were direct quotations from me. Collins told
me later that he did this so that the article would be, as he said, "personal-
ized." He closed his article by writing, "So, please Mr. Legislator, take heed
to the pleadings of Dr. Elliott and other university officials for the 'long
green' that stands in the way right now of giving Texas one of the nation's
leading dental schools and what the school needs is that $2.5 million appro-
priation. That's all." Many used his story to convince the legislators they
called upon. Collins's article was certainly a sight for sore eyes for both Lee
and me since he had used the two illustrations of the cancer hospital and the
dental branch buildings in his article.

In the meantime, plans for other buildings in the Medical Center were
being studied. An architectural firm had been employed to develop plans for
the Medical Center outpatient clinic and for the Institute of Geographic
Medicine. On January 30, Dr. Bertner announced that the building for the
outpatient clinic would be started in about six months at a cost of approximately $2.5 million. Roy Cullen had promised funds for this building and

the architectural firm of Johnson and Maddox had been employed as the architects. The Thomas F. Ellerbe Company of St. Paul, Minnesota, who developed the preliminary plans, was retained as a consultant. Dr. Bertner explained the purpose of the building, which was to serve all the institutions in the Medical Center. In his remarks to the board of trustees he also explained how the clinic would be staffed and how it would operate. Dr. Bertner explained again that the clinic would be under the control and operation of the trustees of the Medical Center. Also, the Medical Center would be responsible for the operating expenses. The staff would comprise faculty members from Baylor University College of Medicine, the University of Texas Dental Branch, the University of Texas School of Public Health, and staff members from all hospitals in the Medical Center that were operating at the time. As other hospitals were completed, their staffs would be appointed to the clinical staff. "As a time saver," Dr. Bertner said, "a pneumatic tube system will be included that will connect all institutions in the center." This was for the purpose of distributing histories of patients and other information that might be needed, as well as a means of communication between the departments in the teaching institutions.

The planned building would be twelve stories. However, in the beginning it would be only four stories, with the foundation constructed to accommodate eight additional floors. The architects' rendition of the plan showed the four-story building and then the later plan with the eight stories added. The twelve-story picture was released later to the newspapers for publication. Dr. Chauncey Leake, after he arrived in Galveston, had decided that the Institute of Geographic Medicine should be located somewhere other than in Houston. In a letter to George Hill he suggested that it might be better if it were located in San Antonio. At the time I thought Dr. Leake might have made this suggestion to offset a circulating rumor that San Antonio was planning to establish a medical school there. On February 10, 1949, an article did appear in the San Antonio papers announcing that a bill had been introduced in the legislature requesting that a medical school be located in San Antonio. This bill was not passed out of committee. However, while it was being considered, it created anxiety for Lee and me. The bill requesting funds for the Houston buildings would not be considered until the San Antonio request had been settled.

Much of the planning done in earlier years was beginning now to bear fruit. While Lee Clark and I worried and waited for the legislature, it was announced on March 7, 1949, that the new Hermann Hospital building had been completed. The new, eight floor building provided Hermann Hospital with four hundred additional hospital beds. This helped to relieve the critical shortage of hospital beds in Houston. This new hospital was the first one to be completed for the Medical Center. The total cost was $5.25 million.

Lee and I were delighted with the way the newspapers throughout the state were helping to support our requests for new building funds. They were adding fuel to our fire by emphasizing that these buildings must be completed at an early date. If one had traveled the long hard road that I had traveled from 1932 to 1949, and the one that Lee had traveled from 1946 to 1949, they could understand why we were so thankful to the large group of prominent citizens from Houston who appeared before the House Budget Committee hearing to support our request for building funds. The group included P. P. Butler, president of the First National Bank and chairman of the chamber of commerce's committee on state and national affairs; Harry Webb, vice president of the Gulf Sulphur Company; Dr. Denton Kerr, president of the Harris County Medical Society; Judge Russell Bonner; Houston Crump, member of the executive committee of the chamber of commerce; and Jesse L. Andrews, assistant vice president of the First National Bank. To me, it was folks like these who were to a large degree responsible for the creation and birth of our Medical Center. Lee and I had been informed by those who were on the Senate Finance Committee and House Appropriations Committee that our bills looked quite favorable and that they would be reported out of the committees with the final note recommending that the bill should pass. Then, on March 29, 1949, Lee and I were startled to read in the papers that another bill for a large appropriation had been introduced in the legislature. It was a sixty million dollar school aid bill. This request, which affected all the school districts in the state, had an abundance of support from schoolteachers, board members, and students who were brought by busloads to Austin.

On the same day, a headline in the *Houston Chronicle* read, "Dental School, Cancer University Unit Cut from Bill." The article explained that the Senate Finance Committee had dropped these two items from the appropriation bill. Of course, I reacted immediately to this announcement because I had been informed of it in advance by Bob Johnson at the time the news came over the wire. Bob had called me because he wanted a rebuttal to the story to be in the same edition. I had it ready. Our story headline, "Fund Loss May Kill Dental School Rating," appeared in the same edition of the *Houston Chronicle,* and it generated considerable heat in Houston and elsewhere throughout the state. The public's reaction to this announcement caused many members of the Senate Finance Committee to react the same way. Bitter complaints came from many senators throughout the state. All of those reactions had an effect. On April 7, an editorial appeared in the *Houston Chronicle* entitled "Fortunately for Texas the Senate Finance Committee is Giving Evidence of Financial Sanity." The editorial was prompted by an announcement made by Senator Taylor, chairman of the Senate Finance Committee. He stated that, "The funds for the University of Texas College of Dentistry and the M. D. Anderson Hospital for Cancer Research should be restored." Probably one of the reasons for this action was that the comptroller for the state, Robert S. Calvert, helped us considerably when he informed the members of the Senate Finance Committee that he would not comply with their requests for an estimate of the cost of the school aid bill. Lee and I began to breathe a little easier. However, from past experience we knew that the appropriation was still not in the bag.

A scrap began between the legislative proponents for our appropriations bill and those opposed to it. Newspapers all over the state took up the fight on our behalf. The pressure brought on by people throughout the state and by the newspapers was terrific. We were heartened over the tremendous support that we were receiving. Yet it was to be a trying time for both Lee and me since other institutions that had budget requests pending were also engaging in the fight. The newspaper stories appeared almost daily. One of the most prominent newspaper articles to appear was in the Greenville *Morning Herald* on April 3, 1949. It was a two-column, front- page editorial entitled, "Our First Duty." To my amazement and happy surprise, the sole purpose of the editorial was to support the Dental Branch building request.

Other requests for funds were disturbing to us. They were for a new medical school in Dallas and for a medical school in San Antonio. This was the second request made by the San Antonio group. These and the school aid bill were just cause for our concern. The Greenville paper read: "It would certainly be a breach of faith if the state did not carry out the obligation it assumed in 1943. A dental school of the first class should be maintained in Texas and the state is already committed to the Houston project . . . we should like to see a state medical school in Dallas, at San Antonio, and other places, but we must not forget that it is our first duty, therefore the first duty of the members of the legislature who represent us, to take care of that which we already have." One of our staunch supporters mailed copies of this editorial to senators all over the state to offset the requests that had been made to them for medical schools in Dallas and San Antonio. This editorial caused quite a stir at the capitol.

The legislature was fast drawing to a close, and still our budget requests had not been considered. Lee and I were waiting anxiously for some action to be taken. On the morning of May 12, the time for rejoicing came once again when it was announced in the morning newspaper that the House had passed the appropriation bill for our two buildings in Houston. However, the Senate had failed to act.[1]

A few days prior to the May meeting of the Medical Center's executive committee, Dr. Bertner discussed the possibility of locating a U.S. Marine Hospital in Houston with Albert Thomas, a congressman from our district. Congressman Thomas suggested to Dr. Bertner that if a tract of ground were allocated in the Medical Center as a site for the hospital, then he would mention this to members of the congressional committee considering the marine hospital. He felt that this might help in getting the committee to give favorable consideration to the bill.

Following Dr. Bertner's remarks, Oveta Culp Hobby suggested that the board should be sure that a marine hospital was needed before this move was made. She informed the board that the Veterans Administration Hospital situation under study as revealed in the Hoover Commission Report, might suggest that it was not needed. Based on Mrs. Hobby's remarks, it was decided that no further discussion concerning this hospital should be held until after the Hoover Commission Report had been published. Later developments confirmed the good judgment of Mrs. Hobby. Also at this meeting, Dr. Bertner read a letter from Dr. Edward Griffey. Dr. Griffey suggested that an eye hospital be established in the Medical Center. At the time, however, an eye, ear, nose, and throat hospital was operating across the street from the Medical Arts Building. Dr. Griffey had indicated in his letter that Mr. Cullen might be interested in building an eye hospital, if the Medical Center would provide a tract of ground for it. The trustees of the Medical Center concluded that this hospital would be too highly specialized and that it should be a part of another hospital. It was Dr. Bertner's opinion that the downtown hospital was all the city needed at the time. Dr. Bertner was requested to inform Dr. Griffey of the action taken. This decision by the trustees confirmed their wisdom. An eye institute was established later at Baylor University College of Medicine and Methodist Hospital provided hospital beds.[2]

In early June the Medical Center's board asked for bids to pave the streets of the Medical Center, as this had not been done yet. H. A. Kipp had planned the streets in the Medical Center so that it would be difficult to use them as traffic ways through the center from Holcombe Boulevard to Fannin Street. At the time, no entrance ways to the Medical Center had been closed. Kipp had designed the streets before planning the tracts of ground. This accounts for the different shapes the tracts of ground had. Later, the traffic between the institutions and traffic entering the Medical Center increased to such an extent that the traffic circle at the Anderson Boulevard intersection became a hazard. It was removed in 1955. Still, the narrow streets that were planned to prevent the flow of traffic through the Medical Center became a severe handicap, even though the streets were used only for Medical Center traffic. Since ground-level parking became overcrowded, it was eventually necessary to provide a number of garages to meet the demands for parking space.

On July 20, 1949, a newspaper article announced that another large gift had been given by the Cullens that would benefit the Medical Center. The gift, announced by Mayor Oscar Holcombe, was a $1.5 million grant to the city of Houston for the construction of a new city-county hospital if the hospital were built in the Medical Center. When the city-county hospital was completed in the Medical Center, the Jefferson Davis Hospital would be converted to a tuberculosis hospital. This plan was Roy Cullen's original idea. The trustees of the Medical Center welcomed the announcement and also his idea for converting the Jefferson Davis Hospital to a tuberculosis hospital. The conversion would allow the trustees to release a tract of ground that was being held in the Medical Center for the construction of the tuberculosis hospital. Cullen's grant would hasten the day when the badly needed city-county hospital could begin construction. The location of the Jefferson Davis Hospital on a spacious lot west of downtown was ideal for a tuberculosis hospital. The Medical Center needed a large teaching hospital, but a tuberculosis hospital did not have to be located in the same area. As Mayor Holcombe observed, "This is a wonderful thing." Roy Cullen said, "The entire future of the Medical Center depends upon the city's participation. Without it the Center can't survive. City cooperation is a must." Difficulties would later arise after Mayor Holcombe made this announcement.

In mid-1949, a feature written by George Fuerman, one of Houston's most colorful feature-story writers, appeared in the morning paper. The story was prompted by the favorable reception that the *Cancer Bulletin* had received from the members of the medical profession. Around 18,000 copies were printed for the first issue of the *Cancer Bulletin* in March, 1948. By mid-1949, the circulation had increased to 61,000. The editor expected that it would grow to over 135,000 by its second birthday. This rather phenomenal growth of a highly specialized journal caused George Fuerman to write about how its editor, Dr. Russell Cumley, had decided to come to Houston. Fuerman wrote:

Dr. Russell Cumley, prior to coming to the Medical Center, was editor of a mid-western medical magazine. . . . However, he always wanted a job in his native state. Dr. Lee Clark had gone to an agency office (available medical personnel agency). He asked them to find someone who might wish to help him develop a cancer publication. Later, the agency called at his hotel and informed him that they had located a person whom they believed would meet Dr. Clark's specifications. Dr. Clark went to the agency office where he found Dr. Cumley waiting for him. Was this a surprise! Dr. Cumley was a boyhood friend of Dr. Clark's back home in Texas. They had not met each other since then. This meeting called for a very long session, until 4 A.M. the next morning, for them to catch up on the past and to talk about the future. Dr. Cumley resigned from his Chicago job just hours later and within a week he was at his desk in Houston as executive-editor of a magazine to be called the *Cancer Bulletin.*

Dr. Cumley retired as editor of the *Cancer Bulletin* in 1975 to devote part of his time to writing about matters dear to his heart. Dr. Cumley would be regarded throughout Texas as one of the most gifted and talented writers in the state.[3]

It was in this year, on December 13, 1949, that ground was broken for the new Methodist Hospital. The spading was done by Bishop Frank A. Smith, with Mr. Walter Goldson, Mrs. W. W. Fondren, and Mrs. Josie Roberts as "overseers." Conversation following the groundbreaking prompted Bishop Smith to reminisce about why the Methodist Hospital was first located at Rosalie and San Jacinto. He said it was located in a small building as a private hospital operated by Dr. O. L. Norseman. Bishop Smith said Norsemen turned it over to Methodist for a nominal sum with the understanding that it would be expanded. Late in 1920, a structure was acquired that Methodist Hospital would occupy until the new building was finished in the Medical Center. I became familiar with this hospital when I first met Josie Roberts at some of the board meetings of social agencies in Houston. Even though the hospital required all of Josie Roberts' working day, she always found time to help in those activities that needed her experienced guidance. She gave her time to the Visiting Nurses Association, the Girl's Home School, and many others. At that time, many of Houston's prominent physicians were on the staff of Methodist Hospital. Among those were Dr. Charles Green, Dr. M. L. Gray, Dr. Joe Poster, and later Dr. J. Charles Dixon.[4]

During the Christmas recess at the Dental Branch, we were preparing for what would be another busy legislative year. Governor Shivers had called a special legislative session to convene on January 31, 1950. It was called so that the legislature could consider many of the budget requests made in the last session that they had failed to act upon. Citizens throughout the state were unhappy with the performance of the last legislature. Many of the budget requests were for Houston projects, therefore Governor Shivers asked Jesse Jones to suggest a group of Houston citizens to serve on a special committee to study the requests and make recommendations to him. Jones suggested Gus Wortham; Dr. E. W. Bertner; Craig Cullinan; former Governor Hobby, *Houston Post* president; George Carmack, editor of the *Houston Press;* and M. E. Walter, editor of the *Houston Chronicle.* The report of this special committee was submitted to Governor Shivers during the early part of January. Their report served as a guideline that the governor used when he presented his message to the opening session of the legislature on January 31, 1950. Immediately following the opening of the legislature, Lee and I were again appearing before legislative committees and we had both prepared new budget requests. The requests were for more than those that we had made at the last session because of the increase in building and material costs. New studies and estimates had been made by the architects and the engineers concerning costs and both of our building requests were increased a considerable degree. The estimate for the Dental Branch building alone had increased more than $200,000 in one year. Lee and I felt that the continuing increase in building costs would help to convince the legislature that to wait any longer would probably result in the same, or even a higher rate of increase. The architects agreed with us. Lee and I were both grateful for the active support that we once again were receiving from the newspapers throughout the state.[5]

Many of the senators and representatives sought information from Lee and me on each of the trips that we made to Austin and we always went prepared. Ed Rider, reporter in charge of the Austin bureau of the *Houston Chronicle,* in an off-hand discussion with me recalled the many years he had seen me coming to each session of the legislature to be available for spur-of-the-moment inquiries from Harris County legislators and from others. In a story he wrote about our conversations, he said that, to his knowledge, I had been coming to Austin for about fifteen years to "fight" for the needs at my institution. He asked me how many trips I had made to Austin and quoted my answer: "I really don't know, but I registered about 22,000 miles on the odometer of my old Ford car just making trips to Austin." Some of this was done in the years that I had traveled to Austin trying to get the legislature to take over the old dental college as a branch of the university. After 1943, the trips were made in order to get a decent building for it. Rider's article followed a meeting of the Senate and House committees on appropriations and the Senate Finance Committee. The paper read: "Dental College Building First Hurdle Has Been Jumped." This was good news to us, but we wondered how successful would we be when we reached the final one?

While in Austin, I read an article in an Austin newspaper about a gift made to the cancer hospital by Mr. and Mrs. Horace Whittington. They had given one hundred shares of Anderson, Clayton & Company stock to the hospital. News reports like this could be used to support our requests. At home, stories continued to appear in the daily papers about the Medical Center—all good news. As these announcements were made, the stories also emphasized the need for the appropriations to build the university buildings in Houston. Another article of major importance announced that the Anderson Foundation would make a grant of $1.5 million to the city for the city-county hospital to be constructed in the Medical Center provided that the voters approved the pending county bond election. The Anderson Foundation grant was to be added to the $1.5 million that Roy Cullen had previously made to the city with the same "if" attached as that of the Cullen Foundation. The balance of the funds needed for the hospital, which was to cost in excess of six million dollars, was to be provided by the city and by a grant from the federal government. From all of our past experiences, Lee and I felt that there was no city that had hope like our city. There was no such word as failure in the Houstonian's vocabulary. Visitors often commented on the warm friendship and enthusiasm of Houston folks, saying, "Houston is just like a country town." We liked this. No matter how busy the prominent people of Houston were, they were always ready to be helpful to those who asked.

The Texas Medical Center was not the only project in Houston that was receiving attention. The rapid growth of the city made it necessary that frequent bonds be issued. The voters had to approve these bond issues and, since Houston was a prosperous city, had not refused any of the requests. All of this prompted Colonel Bates to remark in one of his addresses when calling for action by the legislature that "Houston pays the largest amount in taxes of any city in the state of Texas, but we have only just recently acquired some University of Texas projects. Yet funds are needed for the new buildings if the purposes for which they were created are to serve the citizens of Texas best."

The University of Texas was making rapid progress with its institutions that were located throughout the state. These included Texas Western College in El Paso, the Medical Branch in Galveston, Southwestern Medical College in Dallas, the Dental Branch, the M. D. Anderson Hospital and Tumor Institute in Houston, and the Mc Donald Observatory in West Texas. All of these entities were becoming too much of a load for the president of the university to oversee, as well as to administer the rapidly increasing growth of the large university campus in Austin. At the February meeting of the board of regents, a chancellorship for the university was created. The chancellor would oversee all of the university's widespread activities. Two persons had been mentioned for the chancellorship. One was Dudley Woodward, Jr., chairman of the board of regents, and the other was Hines H. Baker, the former chairman of the university's development board and president of the Humble Oil Company. Both of these gentlemen expressed their appreciation, but declined the invitation. Later, Judge James P. Hart was chosen as the first chancellor of the University of Texas.

The special session of the legislature was rapidly drawing to a close and still no action had been taken on the two bills pending for the Anderson hospital and the Dental Branch. Once again gloom hovered over our heads. Lee and I worked harder than ever—many more tiring hours of waiting on call in Austin for any member of the House or Senate who might need information. Carl Hardin waited with us during the daily sessions. So many bills had been introduced that sufficient funds were not available for all of them. Therefore, each member of the house was jockeying to keep his bill on the docket. Two Harris County legislators, Senator Searcy Bracewell and Representative Bob Casey, introduced separate bills to increase funds through new taxes. Senator Bracewell's bill proposed that a one cent increase in the cigarette tax be added, which he said would provide for buildings in Houston. This bill was not considered. The bill introduced by Bob Casey proposed a long-range program to provide only for building requests made at each legislative session. His bill provided that funds collected from delinquent taxes would be set aside for this purpose. This bill, too, failed. Hope was fading fast.

Then, in the closing hours of the legislature, a joint meeting of the House and Senate appropriations committees was held. Lee and I had been informed of this meeting earlier. As usual, we were waiting outside the senate chamber. We had waited quite some time when Senator Bracewell came out of the meeting to talk with Lee and me. As he approached, I noticed that his expression revealed that all was not well. His statement was forthright. He said that there were not sufficient funds left in the omnibus bill and in the cigarette tax bill to cover both of our requests, but there were sufficient funds for one. Senator Bracewell said he saw no way but to split the money between the cancer hospital and the Dental Branch. This left us in a bind. Neither of us could start a building. The total amount was not even sufficient to cover the building costs of the Dental Branch, and Lee needed less funds. We both would need to wait until the next session to get sufficient funds to complete both buildings if we split the sum of money that Senator Bracewell said was available. I spoke up quickly and suggested that if Bracewell could get the committee to appropriate the full sum for the cancer hospital building then the Dental Branch would wait until the next session. This was, to me, the right way to move and it turned out later that it was. My statement pleased Lee, and Senator Bracewell breathed a sigh of relief. The story in the newspaper the next day reported that the dental school would have to wait until the next session of the legislature.[6]

By then, I had been conditioned to wait. I was ready to try again, though, and preparations for the next session of the legislature immediately began. On March 2, 1950, Governor Shivers signed the $1.35 million appropriation bill for the cancer hospital. While doing so he said, "This is one of the best investments the state has ever made." How true this remark was. Our Medical Center neighborhood was growing rapidly. Many new enterprises were being started and new buildings built nearby. New office buildings, motels, and other businesses appeared across the street from the Medical Center. All of these enterprises served the employees and the visitors who came to the Medical Center.

In 1950, the Prudential Insurance Company of New York announced a new building that was to be constructed in Houston on a site near the Medical Center. No one would have thought at that time that the magnificent structure, which was to be built on Holcombe Boulevard, later would become another building for the University of Texas in our Medical Center. The Cancer Foundation was to be the prime mover in bringing this about. As one may surmise, this was another bit of foresight on the part of Lee. Of course, it was a long time after the announcement was made before the building was constructed for the insurance company.

In March, we were pleased to learn that William Fuerman of Beeville, Texas had willed $250,000 to the cancer hospital. The city of Houston was not forgetting the rapid expansion of the Medical Center and the growth in its vicinity, either. Fannin Street ended at the Warwick Hotel. A short street had been constructed to connect Fannin Street with Main Street. It was not too long after construction began in the Medical Center that the city extended Fannin Street southward. The city engineer recommended this, and the extension was constructed in such a way that it allowed for a three-lane flow of traffic in both directions. At the time, it was considered to be quite adequate for the flow of traffic to the Medical Center and to the growing enterprises to the south. But both Fannin and Main Streets would eventually become crowded.

In June, the University of Houston announced the beginning of the training program at the nursing school in the Medical Center. Included in the program would be a School of Practical Nursing, the first such school in the South. At the time, seventy-seven students were in attendance and the school had been accredited in the latter part of May. The hospital training was done at Hermann, Methodist, and Jefferson Davis Hospitals. Only 112 other practical nursing schools were operating in the United States.

Another first for the Medical Center originated at the Dental Branch. While on a business trip to New York, Dr. Clark learned of the work of Dr. L. B. Vateression, who was using the usual dental prosthetic procedures for restoring parts of the face and head that had to be removed during the surgical treatment of cancer. When Dr. Clark returned to Houston, he suggested to me that we try to get Dr. Vateression to join our Dental Branch faculty. Dr. Vateression accepted our invitation and a maxillofacial prosthetic service was started. At the time, its function was to serve the cancer hospital only. While Dr. Vateression left the Dental Branch some time ago, the maxillofacial prosthetic department has expanded into new facilities provided in M. D. Anderson's rehabilitation hospital. This hospital had formerly been the Southern Pacific Hospital, but was given to the M. D. Anderson Hospital.

The trustees of Methodist Hospital announced that the cornerstone for the building of the new hospital would be laid on May 31, 1950. Dr. E. W. Bertner was the principal speaker. In his address, Dr. Bertner paid tribute to the trustees of Methodist Hospital for having met the challenge of Roy Cullen and the Anderson Foundation in matching the $1 million gift from Cullen and the $500,000 gift from the Anderson Foundation. I was present to hear Dr. Bertner deliver his address. He did so ably and with enthusiasm.[7]

I had a profound admiration for Dr. Bertner. This address, which turned out to be his last public speaking appearance, was a magnificent triumph for him. Many months earlier, Dr. Bertner had mentioned to me an injury he had received to his leg at his country place, just west of Houston. Several weeks later, I noticed that he was rubbing his leg while sitting at the conference table following a meeting of the board of trustees. I asked, "Is your leg still bothering you?" and when he replied "yes," I suggested that he should see a physician. Months passed as Dr. Bertner's full schedule caused him to delay visiting a doctor. Later, specimen studies of the lump he had been rubbing were positive for cancer, and the fight was on. Despite a courageous battle, Dr. Bertner died on July 28, 1950. A great man was gone; a victim of cancer. The glowing tributes paid to Dr. Bertner by the newspapers could not equal those felt in the hearts of his friends. Lee and I had lost a wonderful friend. His death emphasized to me that early detection was half the battle toward curing cancer. Dr. Bertner's death was a great loss to the Medical Center to and all of Texas.[8]

During the fall, Dr. Jack Ewalt, former administrator of the Galveston hospitals that were part of the Medical Branch, became dean of the University of Texas Postgraduate School of Medicine in Houston. He replaced the very busy Dr. Lee Clark who had been serving as acting dean until this appointment could be filled by a full-time dean. Dr. Ewalt, in the short time that he was in the position, developed many activities for the postgraduate school. However, his abilities in the broad field of health resulted in another career step when he was appointed Commissioner of Health for the state of Massachusetts. Once again, Dr. Clark was called upon to assume the duties of acting dean while the search began again for another qualified person for the deanship.

At long last it was announced on September 15 that construction would begin on the new cancer hospital, nine years after Arthur Cato had introduced the bill that created the cancer hospital for Texas. Also, the board of regents had authorized the architects, MacKie and Kamrath, to proceed with the working drawings for the Dental Branch. The board of regents considered it advisable to have the plans ready so that construction could start without delay when the appropriation was made. Some of the regents conjectured that if the appropriation was made in January, 1951, construction for the Dental Branch could begin around March 1, 1951. The regents also announced that an additional request for $1.5 million would be made to provide funds for an additional 100,000 square feet for the cancer hospital. The action taken by the board of regents caused all of us at the Dental Branch to look to the future with renewed vigor and effort.

In October, the Medical Center was fortunate in obtaining the services of another great Houstonian—J. S. Abercrombie had accepted an appointment to the board of trustees of the Children's Hospital. Abercrombie had been one of the founders of the hospital and was largely responsible for its development. Each year for many years Abercrombie's Pin Oak Stables were used for the Pin Oak Annual Charity Horse Show. The show became quite

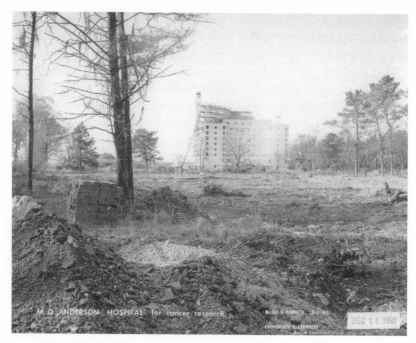

M. D. Anderson Hospital for Cancer Research under construction in the Texas Medical Center, December 14, 1950. Surveyors occasionally encountered rattlesnakes and water moccasins in the wooded area that became the Medical Center.

famous throughout the United States, and the proceeds were contributed to the Texas Children's Foundation for the Children's Hospital. The Houston spirit continued, like a spark, generating many services for the public good as exemplified by Mr. Abercrombie. The Texas Children's Hospital Board of Trustees is but another example of this magnificent spirit. The board members, including J. S. Abercrombie, William A. Smith, Leopold L. Meyer, Lamar Fleming, Herman P. Pressler, Herman Brown, James A. Elkins, Jr., J. W. Leake, Jr., and Wesley W. West, were responsible for the Children's Hospital becoming one of the finest children's hospitals in the United States.

The year closed with the groundbreaking for the new cancer hospital in the Texas Medical Center. This was a happy, long-awaited moment, not only for Lee Clark and his co-workers, but also for the entire city of Houston, the Texas Medical Center, and the University of Texas. As I sat in the little folding chair waiting for the ceremonies to begin, a wee thought of resentment came into my mind. I thought, "I have waited for this day to come for the dental school since 1932 and still it has not come to pass. Then a young man comes to Houston in 1946, and now it is only 1950, and here he is breaking ground." And then I remembered that when I had lamented the same thing to Dr. Painter a few days earlier, he had smiled slightly and said, "Fred, cancer just has more sex appeal than teeth." A smile crossed my face, and I forgot my resentment. I, too, would have my day, but for now I was to have only good thoughts. December 20, 1950, was indeed Christmas Day for Lee Clark. Though each year that would pass after this day was filled with some new accomplishment for Lee, none could bring the joy of complete fulfillment to him that this one had brought. It was his first "red wagon" and there were many more to come.[9]

CHAPTER 6

A New Era
Executive Director of the Texas Medical Center

AS WE BEGAN 1951, many new projects were launched at the Texas Medical Center. Each day the sound of saws, hammers, riveters, bulldozers, and other noise-making devices greeted visitors to the center. These sounds were not just noise to some of us. It was music, in all its cacophony. New institutions were buzzing with activity. Research on polio was going forward at Baylor. A new postgraduate teaching program began at the newly established University of Texas Graduate School of Biomedical Science. Dr. S. S. Arnim, who had joined the Dental Branch faculty much earlier, was appointed dean of the new school in February, 1951. A new addition was announced for the already completed Veterans Administration Hospital. It was to cost a "mere" three million dollars.

The year started on a glad note. A crippled child with a happy face helped to lay the cornerstone of the new Shrine Crippled Children's Clinic and Hospital. In his remarks as principal speaker for this occasion, John H. Freeman said, "In this clinic children are treated without cost and without any distinction as to color or creed or race." It also was announced that two hospitals located elsewhere in the city were to become teaching hospitals for the Postgraduate School of Medicine of the University of Texas. These hospitals, the Southern Pacific Hospital and St. Joseph's Hospital, were two of the oldest in Houston. They had been serving the community for many years both for charity as well as for other patients. Southern Pacific Hospital was an annex of the Anderson Hospital and also served as a rehabilitation center for patients who had been treated at the cancer hospital. The hospital was given to the University of Texas as a gift from the Southern Pacific Railroad. The beds in the hospital were for the ambulatory patient who must be confined in a hospital while under treatment. Many beds in the M. D. Anderson Hospital, which were formerly used for this purpose, were freed for the more critically ill patient.[1]

In the early part of 1951, Lee Clark had the opportunity to present the Bertner Award for Cancer Research to a friend of his, Dr. Fred Stuart,

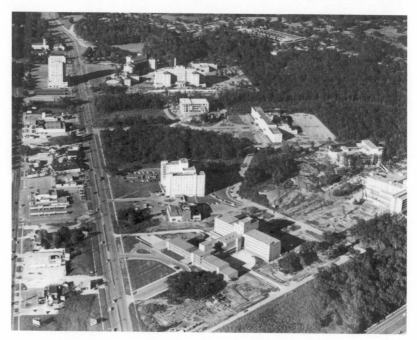

Texas Medical Center construction, 1953. Courtesy Texas Medical Center

pathologist at Memorial Hospital in New York. This was to be the first award in Dr. Bertner's honor since his death. Dr. Stuart paid a warm tribute to Dr. Bertner, whom he had known for several years. At the same time, Chancellor Hart presented a Jesse H. Jones Scholarship to Dr. E. C. Hinds, who at the time was professor of oral surgery at the Dental Branch. Dr. Hinds completed his scholarship at the M. D. Anderson Hospital, after which he passed his board in general surgery. Dr. Hinds had completed his degree in dentistry and medicine at Baylor University. His father was dean of Baylor University College of Dentistry in Dallas. He would have been proud of his son on that day had his death some time earlier not intervened.

My warm regard and great admiration for Governor Shivers continued to grow. His first recommendation for providing funds for the Dental Branch building was made in his opening address before the joint session of the legislature. His remarks were heart warming. His personal interest in the dental school was demonstrated again on April 20, in a newspaper headline that read: "Shivers Renews Plea for Dental School Funds." One of Governor Shivers's remarks in the article reminded the legislature that he had asked for this appropriation in his opening address. On May 5, 1951, with the closing of the legislative session drawing near, our long and continued prayers were answered. An *Austin American-Statesman* headline announced: "Houston's Long Sought Dental School Building Has Been Given the Green Light in the 1951–53 Appropriation Bill." The article said that the state would provide $2,365,000 for the new building. Governor Shivers time and again demonstrated the faith that the voters had in him when they made him governor for the second time. Allan Shivers continued to grow in stature, into one of Texas' "imminent own" by continuing to expand his life in services to the people of Texas. My often-repeated remark was, "Governor Shivers is the kind of man we need for president."

Our emotions were torn in two directions when we learned that Dr. Walter H. Scherer had died on the same day that the appropriation bill passed. Though deeply grieved, we added to our prayers of thankfulness for this day, May 5, prayers of thankfulness for his patient and untiring support during the twenty preceding years. Dr. Scherer did not forget us—his will stipulated that seventy-five thousand dollars be given to the University of Texas for the Dental Branch. Ann and I grieved again over the loss of a very dear friend who had meant so much to us during our years in Houston. First and much earlier, Dr. Finis Hight, and now Walter Scherer. It was a saddened, yet glad day.

Later in May, the physicians who had started much earlier toward their dreams for a children's hospital in the Medical Center had reason to celebrate. On May 18, 1951, a contract was signed with the Tellepsen Construction Company for the construction of the hospital in the Medical Center. Many prominent Houstonians had rallied behind the physicians in their desire to bring about this happy day. Those present at the time the contract was signed included Leopold Meyer, chairman of the board of trustees of the hospital; Howard Tellepsen, president of the construction company; R. H. Abercrombie; J. S. Abercrombie; and Jesse H. Jones. On May 24, groundbreaking ceremonies were held for the Children's Hospital. Dr. Russell H. Blattner, professor of pediatrics and head of the department of pediatrics at Baylor University College of Medicine, was appointed chief-of-staff of the hospital. He was one of the speakers for the groundbreaking exercises.[2]

A short time later on June 13, 1951, Dr. Lee Cady, administrator of the veterans hospital, announced that a contract had been let to the Farnsworth and Chamber's Construction Company for the new $2,182,900 addition to the hospital. This new addition was to be the neuropsychiatric unit for the Veterans Administration Hospital and construction would begin in the fall. The neuropsychiatric unit would become a valuable teaching facility for Baylor College of Medicine.

In July, one of Houston's colorful figures, Glen McCarthy, standing in for

Walter Winchell (treasurer for the David Runyon Memorial Fund), presented a check to Lee Clark for twenty-five thousand dollars. This sum was applied to the cost of research that was needed for the development of the Cobalt-60 Irradiator, which was being conducted by Dr. Grimmett and Dr. Gilbert Fletcher. The Cobalt-60 unit would become the first one in the United States.

In September, Earl Hankamer, president of the Prudential Oil Company, was elected to the board of trustees of the Texas Medical Center. Hankamer was chairman of the board of trustees of Arabia Crippled Children's Clinic and Hospital, a member of the board of trustees of Hermann Hospital, and vice president of the executive committee of Baylor College of Medicine. He was to fill the place left vacant by Ray Dudley, who had been an active and tireless worker both for Baylor and the Medical Center before he died.[3]

Another first for the Medical Center occurred when the new Speech and Hearing Center opened on September 15, 1951. W. T. Sutherland, president of the Henke-Pillot Grocery Company and a member of the board of trustees of the Speech and Hearing Center, had invited Dr. J. L. Bangs to Houston to discuss an appointment as director of the center. Dr. Bangs, who had been a professor of the speech and hearing clinic at the University of Washington, accepted the appointment. Methodist Hospital provided space for the Speech and Hearing Center, which was to serve children in the same manner as the Shrine Crippled Children's Clinic. Any child who had speech and hearing difficulties was to be treated in the clinic regardless of race, creed, color, or financial state. Individual donors and the community chest provided funds for those who could not pay. A short time later, Tina Bangs, Dr. J. L. Bangs's wife, joined him as a coworker in the clinic and eventually became director. Today, a large and magnificent building houses the Speech and Hearing Center. It has become a teaching and research unit of the University of Texas and is staffed by members of the faculty of the University of Texas Medical School and others.

Many groups interested in health were engaged in activities that added to the development of the Medical Center, but none of the groups were more helpful than the Junior League of Houston. Their interest in the welfare of children was legion. They went forward with their activities in a quiet, unassuming manner, providing funds for many different children's projects. They also gave their time to institutions with childcare programs. In October, 1951, it was announced that the Junior League was to enlarge its scope of work at Hermann Hospital. The Junior League program at Hermann Hospital had started in 1944. However, the Junior League started their first activities in a children's clinic and health center for children in the First National Bank Building in 1947. They provided the clinic with a full-time pediatrician, a full-time secretary, and a Junior League volunteer each day. Now they were to have the opportunity to be of even greater service in the newly expanded children's clinic at Hermann Hospital. Not only were they providing funds to Baylor Medical College and to Hermann Hospital to help defray expenses for the clinic, but they also were to serve personally as volunteers for office, clinic, and ward duty. Twenty-seven provisionals were assigned to these duties. These young ladies made personal sacrifices and were very much appreciated. They had much to do with the financing of the new Children's Hospital building, and their work has not stopped yet.

As the end of the year drew near, another spade of dirt was turned and another hospital for the Medical Center was on its way. On September 28, 1951, Bishop Quin and Roy Cullen, with his rector, the Reverend Smith of Palmer Memorial Church, each wielded a spade for the groundbreaking ceremonies for St. Luke's Hospital. Yet another proud day was to follow shortly. On November 11, the dedication exercises for the new Methodist Hospital and the Weiss Memorial Chapel, named for Harry C. Weiss's mother, were held. The chapel was a gift provided by the Weiss family in memory of Harry Weiss who died in 1948. He was one of the founders and had served as president of the Humble Oil and Refining Company. Thus another year closed and just as they had done in the previous year, Methodist pulled down the shade.

As in 1951, we heralded another year of exciting events in 1952. Some we knew would occur; others would be a surprise. Interesting announcements began early in the year. The Academy of Medicine announced on January 8, that it had approved the plans for the new Academy of Medicine library, which would cost $1.2 million. Then on January 21, J. S. Abercrombie and Leopold Meyer proudly exhibited a brochure that Walt Disney had prepared for them. The little Disney characters were asking for funds to help build the Texas Children's Hospital. This was a generous gesture from the man I had known in Kansas City who, at that time, could have given his time, but had little else to give.

On January 28, the University of Texas Board of Regents stopped in Houston on their way to Galveston for a board meeting. Their stop was to allow three members to visit our Medical Center: Tom Sealy of Midland, Claude Voyle of Austin, and Dr. L. S. Oates of Center. The older members of the board were happy with the manner in which their early efforts were being rewarded. Construction was underway for the new neuropsychiatric building at the veterans hospital. One of the items on the docket was the final plan for the Dental Branch building. On February 1, the regents announced that they would ask for bids for this new building about March 26, 1952. The architects had estimated the cost to be about $6.45 million. The students at the Dental Branch were pleased by this announcement. They had literally sweated it out in the old dental school building. To attend classes in a non-air-conditioned building in a Texas July was something that most of them would not forget.[4]

The new Shrine Crippled Clinic and Children's Hospital opened on February 16, 1952. It was a special day for John Freeman and many others who had worked long and hard for this day to arrive. What a day it was for Geneva Ann Wright, the little girl who was at the groundbreaking exercises for the hospital in a wheelchair. She had held the spade when the first shovel of dirt was turned. For opening day, the wheelchair was gone and she cut the ribbon—quite an occasion for this seven-year-old girl.

On the same day, Dr. Gilbert Fletcher appeared in the newspaper pictured with a full-size model of the Cobalt-60 Irradiator, which he helped design. An imitation specimen of a small piece of cobalt was shown in its tiny steel box, about an inch square. This same size piece of real cobalt-60 would have "more radioactive strength than the world's entire supply of radium." Another first for the Medical Center. The Texas Medical Center was a place where scientists with vision wanted to be. Many like Dr. Gilbert Fletcher, who was from Paris, France, came from far and wide. He would become surrounded by many more powerful tools than the one he demonstrated on that day in 1952.

Finally, on May 3, 1952, *the* day arrived. May 3 was a day that brought thanksgiving and joy to many hearts at the Dental Branch and throughout the state. This day was to be the groundbreaking day for the new Dental Branch building. By their appropriation, the legislature had provided the total amount that was needed for the construction of our building. The Anderson Foundation previously had provided us with an additional grant, which allowed us to proceed with our building as planned. It would not be necessary to ask for more.

We were blessed with a beautiful day, and a large group of over five hundred citizens was there to congratulate every person who had so much to do with bringing this occasion about. Yet, looking back, I rather feel that this large group was actually congratulating each other. It seemed that all of them had played an important part in making this day possible. As one could expect, I felt very proud to look about and see so many friends on the platform to congratulate us. Our guests included Chancellor Hart; Mayor Oscar Holcombe; Marvin Hurley, vice president and general manager of the chamber of commerce; James Rockwell, the Houston member of the board of regents; State Senator Searcy Bracewell; John Freeman, vice president of the M. D. Anderson Foundation; and Dr. Marcus Murphy, president of the Houston District Dental Society. They were there not only to speak on behalf of the institutions they represented, but also because each of them had done so much to help the university establish a dental school for the people of Texas. They had also kept the legislative bodies from forgetting that this was a project that they, the taxpayers, wanted done. The members of the legislature—almost one and all, heartily agreed. Each one who spoke had something nice to say about everyone else except themselves. Chancellor Hart and I both expressed deep appreciation to the Anderson Foundation, whose gift of $1.25 million was the largest single gift ever made to a dental school up to that date except for one other large gift that had been given by Montgomery Ward to Northwestern University for their dental school. Likewise, Chancellor Hart and I thanked the chamber of commerce for the large part they had played through many years, from 1931 to that day in 1952, in helping the dental college to become a part of the university. We also expressed appreciation for their fund drive for the university buildings in the Medical Center as well as for Baylor College of Medicine, our sister institution.

Folding chairs had been provided in front of the platform for the number of visitors that we thought would attend. There were far too few. One of the chairs in the front row was occupied by Elna Birath, who was overcome with emotion almost throughout the entire proceedings. I glanced her way many times with an unspoken "thank you" on my lips. I had wanted her to be on the platform, but she had refused. She said, "If I were there, everyone from the dental school should be there too." She was right. But she knew that I knew that this day of celebration might not have been possible had she not insisted that I remain with the dental college during a bleak time when I had wanted to resign. Of course, behind those seated in the audience was a large group who waited—our students, faculty, and the staff who had done so much. Among all of them, none could have been prouder than Mr. Loock, who was in charge of maintenance for our dental school, and his two staunch helpers. One of them, Jack Johnson, had been with us since the time I arrived in Houston. I made it a point to go over to this group after the ceremony and thank them for what they had done to bring this day about. I also thanked the few remaining students—many had left to go back to work, even though it was a day off for them.[5]

In the first part of May, we were saddened by the untimely death of J. M.

Jackson, assistant treasurer of the Medical Center. I had worked with him from the beginning of our Medical Center to the time of his death. It was sad news for the members of our board and also to the members of the board of trustees of the Anderson Foundation. He had served as secretary of the M. D. Anderson Foundation for quite some time. Jackson and I were fellow Rotarians. His wife had been the prime moving force behind the early development of the Rotary-Anns and served as their first president. Her interest in the Dental College for many years before it became a part of the university was largely responsible for the successful orthodontic program that was established. The Rotary-Ann Clinic still continues to serve underprivileged children of Houston.

Later in the month, we learned that Dr. Mavis P. Kelsey, who had taken time out from a busy practice to serve as acting dean of the postgraduate school, would soon be relieved of this extra task. On June 1, Dr. Roscoe Pullen arrived to assume his duties as dean of the University of Texas Postgraduate School of Medicine. The board of regents had appointed him at their meeting in March. Dr. Pullen was leaving his post as vice-dean of Tulane University School of Medicine to come to the Medical Center.[6]

The end of another school year was approaching. I have mentioned that the Cobalt-60 Irradiator was to be the first unit of its type in the M. D. Anderson Hospital. Now on July 23, 1952, M. D. Anderson announced the acquisition of a new Betatron unit, a super x-ray machine. It was a 24 million-volt machine, and though it was hard to believe, Dr. Gilbert Fletcher said it was eight times stronger than the Cobalt-60 Irradiator. This was another first for our Medical Center.

The sounds of hammers and saws and belching bulldozers continued while the constant up and down movement of material lifts seemed to never cease. During the year, four buildings were under construction, with the possibility of two more to start. The Medical Center was a busy place. Houston, the fastest-growing city in the nation according to the newspapers [600,000 people], continued to grow. The Medical Center, with millions of building dollars flowing in, along with the expenditures of students, teachers, patients, and others, added to the continued prosperity of the city.

In August, the architects' preliminary sketches of the new city-county hospital for the Medical Center were published in the daily papers. It was to be a large, beautiful building estimated to cost sixteen million dollars, a rather huge sum in 1952. Some time earlier, the Medical Center had acquired land adjacent to the Shrine Crippled Children's Clinic and Hospital. They attained it from the city in a trade for a tract of ground located at the south-east corner of the Medical Center on Holcombe Boulevard, adjoining Braes Bayou to the east.

That summer, two well-prepared black students were admitted to the dental school's freshman class. They were our first black students, but only because none had previously applied. One of these students went on to be an instructor at the Dental Branch of the University of Texas. Many other black students have graduated from Medical Center schools since these first two were accepted.[7]

Back in 1950, the trustees of the Medical Center had appointed a search committee following Dr. Bertner's death. This committee was to recommend to the trustees someone who could become a full-time director of the Medical Center. During the time that had elapsed, the members of the committee had made many contacts, yet none proved fruitful in finding a director who could fill Dr. Bertner's shoes and who wanted to accept an appointment. One of the members of the committee was Hines Baker. One day, in the early part of September, 1952, just a few months after ground had been broken for our new dental school, my secretary informed me that Baker was on the phone. I was surprised to learn that he had placed this call personally. I answered quickly. Baker then said, "Doctor, we have been searching for a man for the executive-directorship of the Medical Center for some time. We have looked for one who could meet certain requirements we felt were necessary. Well, I have that man." I was eager to know whom he had located. He continued by saying, "I don't know why I had not thought of this before, but the thought just struck me this morning that you are the man to take this place."

I was both amazed and concerned almost simultaneously. I imagine that I stammered somewhat to hear this statement from Hines Baker, but I cannot recall. He went on to say that he felt I had certain qualifications that uniquely fit this position. Before I had time to answer, Baker mentioned the concern that had entered my own mind when he first mentioned all of this to me. The concern was about the dental school. He allayed this feeling somewhat by pointing out that I would be close by to assist the new dean on any occasion that he might need to call upon me. He made the point very strongly that the Medical Center had gone too long without a leader. He explained that none of the trustees, except for me, had time to guide the Medical Center during the period following Dr. Bertner's death. He then asked my permission to discuss this matter with the other trustees. I agreed. I did have a breathing spell, a period during which I confidentially discussed this offer with many faculty members, including Mrs. Birath and with Chancellor Hart. As I expected, all of them expressed keen disappointment and asked that I give the offer prayerful consideration before accepting. At the time, I probably knew better than anyone else the reason behind Baker's concern about the Medical Center. But I also knew that it was a critical time for me to be leaving the dental school. I was confronted with a tough decision. Ann was in the dilemma with me. After considerable time, and many more discussions with those at the dental school, including some of our outstanding students, I made the decision that if I were offered the position as director of the Medical Center, I would accept.

A few days later James Anderson called and asked if I had time to visit with him in his office. A time was set and the meeting was held. I was to become the new head of the Texas Medical Center—a great surprise to the profession, to the people of Houston, and to the people of the state. To them, I had become "Mr. Dental School." Congratulations poured in from everywhere and I have cherished those letters through the years. The chancellor appointed a committee to select a new dean of the Dental Branch and they met with him, during my absence, in my office. They told him that they felt that Dr. John V. Olson was the candidate that they wished to recommend. Prior to this meeting, Chancellor Hart had asked me if I had any suggestions of members of the faculty who might serve as dean. I suggested three members of the faculty that I believed were qualified to serve as the dean; Dr. John V. Olson was one of the three. Dr. Olson, a graduate of the University of Michigan, was a member of the faculty in the department of mouth and facial restorations and served as coordinator of clinical instruction. Chancellor Hart informed Dr. Olson that he had been selected as the new dean of the Dental Branch, effective November 1, 1952.[8]

One of Dr. Bertner's cherished dreams was realized on October 15, when three spades of dirt were turned by his widow, Mrs. Julia Bertner, and by Mrs. Jesse Jones, and Mrs. Claude Cody for the library building groundbreaking. As one reporter expressed it, these were "spades of gold" that they used, for during the ceremony, Dr. Moise Levy announced that Jesse Jones had given $600,000 as a gift to the Academy of Medicine to construct the library building. The Anderson Foundation had previously given $300,000. Physicians, dentists, and friends had given an additional $150,000. Dr. Levy and Dr. Claude Cody had worked long and hard to bring this day about. This was another day for Dr. Bertner since it was he who had tried to provide a library building near Hermann Hospital quite some time before the advent of the Medical Center.[9]

On the morning of November 1, 1952, I walked into the offices of the

Texas Medical Center, the same offices that Dr. Bertner had occupied before his death. They were adjacent to his professional offices. I was greeted warmly by Sue Barnett, who had done so much for the Medical Center as administrative assistant to Dr. Bertner. Her admiration for Dr. Bertner's ability and driving force caused her to serve the center long after she originally told Dr. Bertner that she would help him temporarily. She remained with the Medical Center until she had indoctrinated me with the ongoing daily operations of the office.

As the trustees of the Medical Center had anticipated, I had many immediate problems. I met innumerable times with the administrators of the institutions in the Medical Center, with physicians, the business managers of the institutions, and many members of the board of trustees of each institution. I asked them to make recommendations about immediate matters that needed attention. There were many. The workdays began early in the morning before even arriving at the office and ended many hours after it had closed.

Of course, it was difficult for me to let a day pass without visiting the Dental Branch, which was under construction at the time. I visited the old dental school many times. Dr. Olson had permitted me to keep my laboratory at the Dental Branch, which I used from time to time to continue some projects I had not completed at the time I left the dental school. Dr. Olson was fast settling into his new position and the students and faculty respected their new dean. The job had fallen into his lap literally overnight. It was a difficult situation for him since his previous duties had not required him to follow the details of building construction. In addition to conducting the many local, state, and national business relations and preparing for the opening session of the legislature in 1953, being dean was quite a large order. All of these were confrontations that the average person would not have cared to assume, but Dr. Olson was not average. My misgivings about leaving the school were quickly dispelled. Dr. Olson had assumed command in a masterful fashion, and his coworkers were prepared to help him immensely.

During the latter part of November, the M. D. Anderson Foundation, in addition to their several previous large gifts, made another gift of $1.2 million to the M. D. Anderson Hospital for the construction of an additional wing. This wing was to be known as the Bertner Memorial Wing. The Anderson Foundation's gift inspired many others to make additional contributions to the hospital for furnishing the new wing. Mr. and Mrs. Nathan Klein, who gave fifty thousand dollars, were among those making larger donations.

Of my various social agency relations from my early years in Houston, I had been a member of the first group that was organized to combat the ravages of polio. On December 31, 1952, Elmer Bertelson wrote a story about public health in Houston during the past year. His first item was one that was to concern Houstonians and was a big concern of the scientists in our Medical Center—the largest polio epidemic in the history of the city. While this announcement was tragic, it served to help generate funds for research in the study of diseases like polio. Baylor's staff of researchers was hard at work on this difficult problem. Also, two months after I had opened the doors to my Medical Center office, Dr. Stanley Olson did likewise at Baylor University College of Medicine. Dr. Walter Moursund had retired, and on January 1, 1953, Olson assumed his duties as the school's new dean. Dr. Olson was to become a dynamic leader in the growth and development of the medical school and the Medical Center.

In early February, members of the legislature were invited to attend a stock show and rodeo in Houston. The chamber of commerce might have had another purpose in mind, since before the legislators were taken to the rodeo, they were first taken on a guided tour through the Medical Center to view what had been accomplished with the appropriations made at three previous legislative sessions. It was hoped that their visit to Houston would remind them that they still faced a responsibility since budget requests from the University of Texas units in the Medical Center had already been introduced. The remarks that some of the representatives made to reporters while visiting the Medical Center seemed to indicate that they were pleased with what they saw. Representative Horace Houston, Jr., of Dallas remarked, "It is a capital investment in the future of the State. If all state money was as well spent, we wouldn't have to worry about a thing." Speaker of the House, Rueben Senterfitt, was especially impressed with having the opportunity to see for the first time the fruit of a bill he had helped to co-sponsor. He was co-author of the bill that created the M. D. Anderson Hospital in 1941.

Representative Bill Daniel of Liberty, one of Texas' truly colorful citizens, called for an unscheduled stop at Methodist Hospital since he was a trustee of the hospital and wanted to see what had been done. He was proud of what he saw. Brief stops were made at Rice Institute, the University of Houston, and then another unscheduled stop at the Prudential Building, a magnificent structure that had just been completed.

The time was approaching for Dr. Mavis Kelsey, who once again had been called upon to serve as interim dean, to present a budget request for the Postgraduate School of Medicine of the University of Texas. This would be the third time that a request had been made for supporting funds. The Anderson Foundation had been supporting the school during the years since it was first established. Now it was time for the state to assume its responsibility. Dr. Kelsey, who was hard at work preparing material to present to the appropriations committee of the legislature, asked many groups in Houston who had previously come forth for this same purpose to help in this endeavor. Among those to help were the medical societies of the state, especially the Harris County Medical Society, the chamber of commerce of Houston, Baylor Medical College, the M. D. Anderson Foundation, the board of regents of the University of Texas, and the trustees of the Medical Center. I prepared material which I thought would be of help to Dr. Kelsey. In a report I had prepared to be read before the House Appropriations Committee I stated: "An appropriation was a necessity for the people of Texas. This school, if supported properly, would provide teaching programs for the practicing physician that would keep him informed on the recent advancements made in medicine." I mentioned further in the report that "residencies in hospitals would be available for those who wished to qualify for a specialty in medicine. Special research projects were to be developed for both medical students and practicing physicians who desired to study in some special field." I closed by stating that "The budget request was a small price for the people of Texas to pay for the benefits that they would receive. Indeed a very low price to pay when compared to other educational costs of lesser importance." Once again, the budget request would be denied.

Now was the time for the heads of the University of Texas institutions in Houston to appear before the various legislative committees held in Austin. They would present their case in support of their budget requests. On the morning of February 26, Dr. Olson, dean of the Dental Branch, with the support of Chancellor Hart, was to make his first appearance before one of the committees. I knew how he felt. One was never quite sure of the inner feelings of the members of the committee at the moment, or how they felt about this or that item in the budget request. Were any of them in a bad mood because of what might have occurred during the previous hearing? Or did they have a bad experience when they last visited their dentist?

Following the hearing for the Dental Branch in the morning, Dr. Clark appeared before the same committee during the afternoon session. Clark made his presentation for approval of his budget, and the headline in the next morning's paper read, "Solons Spellbound by Fight on Cancer." When I read about the session, I was reminded of Dr. Painter's earlier comment about teeth not having the same sex appeal as cancer. The first line of the article read, "Texas Senators listened with rapt attention Wednesday afternoon when Dr. Lee Clark told the dramatic story of the fight against cancer being waged at the M. D. Anderson Hospital in Houston." Senator Crawford Martin of Hillsborough told Dr. Clark that he could "sit here and listen to you talk all afternoon." I believe that if Dr. Painter had been with me at the time I was reading this article, he might have remarked, "See what I mean?"

Just a few days after Representative Bill Daniel visited the Methodist Hospital, a pet project of his in the Medical Center, it was announced that on February 1, 1953, Josie Roberts, the efficient and gracious lady who had conducted his tour, would retire. A large group of Josie's friends and associates were present at the farewell dinner given for her at the Rice Hotel. No one could have served an institution as inspiringly and as devotedly as Josie Roberts had done. She had been with Methodist Hospital since it first opened and served as its administrator for twenty-one years. She had accomplished what she had started out to do—a magnificent new structure now housed her Methodist Hospital. Ted Bowen had worked with her as an assistant administrator during the time that the building was being planned. He was to take her place as administrator of Methodist Hospital. It was a joyous evening for Josie.[10]

Another big day arrived for Lee Clark on March 19, when the cornerstone for his new building was to be laid. Many dignitaries from everywhere were present to help Lee celebrate this grand occasion. Almost all of our university officials were there. Chancellor Hart gave the principal address. The chairman of the board of regents, Tom Sealy of Midland, said, "We see the real, the tangible evidence of how mankind makes progress. Progress is made by men who dream." There was no need now for a "Texas brag" about our Medical Center—others were doing it for us, far and wide, over the mountains and across the oceans. On April 11, twenty doctors from eleven foreign countries visited us. They came to see this "great Medical Center" that they had read about and became the houseguests of seventeen of our Houston physicians. The doctors that visited the Medical Center were from China, Greece, Iran, Portugal, Philippines, Yugoslavia, Italy, and South America. They were tremendously impressed with what they saw and almost overwhelmed when we talked about our dreams for the future. We appreciated their visit.

In May, we prepared to dedicate the opening of a new hospital in the Medical Center. It seemed only yesterday that the groundbreaking was completed, yet the great day had finally arrived. On May 15, 1953, the Texas Children's Hospital was dedicated. Persistence and guided determination had brought this hospital into being. Dr. David Greer and his supporters, who had looked for a listening ear in the early days, could not help but feel happy and proud that now this dream of theirs was a reality. Leopold "Lep" Meyer, J. S. Abercrombie, and many others were there to celebrate, for they, too, had helped make this day possible. Dr. Stanley Olson, the new dean of Baylor University College of Medicine was the principal speaker. I sat with others on stage to listen to a forceful address. Lee Gamm II, the administrator who had guided the planning of the hospital, was on stage, too, and was a happy man. In June we learned that even though he was a very busy man, Gamm had accepted an appointment to the development board of the University of Texas.

In July, a cloud appeared on the horizon for the Medical Center, possibly indicating that a storm was brewing. At the time, we could not have predicted how long this storm might last. Our desire to build the new city-county hospital in our Medical Center would be challenged. The challenge was presented by conscientious, well-meaning men; physicians who were deeply concerned as to whether the move would really benefit those who needed the services of the hospital. It was the belief of these physicians that this hospital, if located in the Medical Center, would be too far from where the patients lived. Pro and con debates started and would continue for some time to come. As time passed during this unfortunate period, the debates became more testy and heated. Many physicians joined with those in favor of the hospital being located in the Medical Center. They did not allow themselves to become blinded by the fears of those who opposed the location. The public remarks that the physicians made in support of the Medical Center location caused some of them to develop enemies within their profession. Like so many occurrences of this type, the misgivings were eventually overshadowed by the good that came out of having the hospital located in the Texas Medical Center. The dire conditions that were predicted did not come to pass. Some of the funds that had been promised for the construction of the hospital had been cancelled when the controversy became quite heated, and it would take some time to restore the confidence of those who were to the provide funds, as well as to convince some members of the public that the Medical Center was the proper location. This cloud, which appeared on the horizon in July, 1953, grew into a storm that lasted weeks, months, and years. Yet, just like the lines of squalls and the hurricanes that visit Houston from time to time but do not prevent the city's forward movement, the Medical Center, too, moved along on its set path.[11]

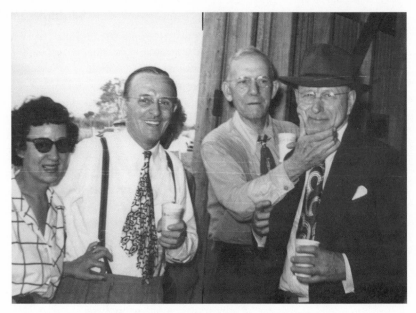

Ann Elliott and Fred Elliott. Courtesy E. W. D'Anton

Later in the month, Governor Shivers appointed Dr. Hampton Robinson, one of Houston's enterprising and promising physicians, to become a member of the State Board of Health. Dr. Robinson was an enthusiastic supporter of our Medical Center and also a member of the faculty of Baylor College of Medicine. Dr. Robinson served many years as president of the State Board of Health, including the period that the board was responsible for the approval of federal grants for hospital construction throughout the state. Because of the rapid growth of Houston, the board made several large grants to Houston hospitals, some of them in the Medical Center. It was not until 1975 that Dr. Robinson resigned from the hospital board. Through his long tenure on the Board of Health, Dr. Robinson continued to serve Baylor College of Medicine in his "without pay" appointment on the faculty.

In the last days of July of the not-to-be-forgotten year of 1953, Ann and I made plans for a few weeks rest in the lake country of Missouri, a boyhood stomping ground. Before leaving on our vacation, I decided to have a minor surgical operation to correct a nagging problem. This was to be done over the weekend and I would to return to the office on Monday morning. I did return on a Monday morning, but during the latter part of September instead of July! An unforeseen circumstance developed that created a serious situation for me. Fortunately, with excellent medical care and prayerful support from hundreds of friends, I did not "leave" as it was feared by some of my physicians and friends. Of course, Missouri had been forgotten.[12]

Just as many of the Medical Center coworkers and I were settling back into work, another concern developed. Horace Wilkins, who had served as a founding member of the Anderson Foundation board and also as a founding member of the Medical Center board, was admitted to Hermann Hospital in critical condition. His illness was of a similar nature to mine. I ran across the street to Hermann Hospital immediately upon learning of his condition. I visited with him several times during his last few days. He died in the latter part of September, less than three weeks after I had returned to the office. It was a sad misfortune for the Medical Center. His long tenure on our board and with the Anderson Foundation had provided us with his guidance in the proper direction many times when some financial difficulty arose. He would be missed.

I had always considered Lee Clark a teammate of mine, but Lee could belong to many other teams without losing interest or affection for any one of the others. He was now a member of a new team: Clark, Cumley, and Klautz. John P. Klautz was head of the Elsevier Press, a publisher of scientific and health information. This team became involved in a tremendous task, which began in the latter part of September. They were to write, edit, and publish *The Book of Health,* a short title for an unlimited subject. I wonder if they had known then that millions of words would be included in this nine hundred-plus page book (with over fourteen hundred illustrations), would they have still tackled the job? I'm sure Lee would have. He had no limit to his endurance.[13]

The year ended on a happy note when Mr. and Mrs. Hugh Roy Cullen gave one million dollars in additional funds to the Baylor University College of Medicine. This was indeed a happy year for us in the Medical Center and for Baylor College of Medicine. On the evening of December 29, Ann and I were present at the Cullen's home, along with many other friends of theirs, to congratulate them on their fiftieth wedding anniversary. It was a joyful day for the Cullens and for all that were present. Ann and I, along with hundreds of others, loved the Cullens.

In November, 1953, Governor Shivers had called a special session of the legislature to meet on January 1, 1954, to consider additional financing for many of the state institutions. During the beginning days of January, the House and Senate floors buzzed with the activities of the legislators. The M. D. Anderson Hospital and the Dental Branch were still short of funds for the final completion of their buildings and for purchasing new equipment. These funds were provided by the new legislature.

We learned on January 12, 1954, that Howard Hughes had made it official. Previously, all of the announcements about the large foundation he was to establish were made as if it were official, but it would prove later not to be the case. This announcement, though, was the first that Hughes had authorized for release. It was explained that he had incorporated the Hughes Medical Institute under the laws of the state of Delaware. Hughes would not discuss the extent of his holdings that he had transferred to the institute, other than to say that the Hughes Aircraft Company was now a subsidiary of the Institute. Hughes hastened to explain that this part of the company was not tax exempt. In the article, Hughes stated that during the past three years he had supported several scholarships and fellowships. The scientists in training were to be available to the institute when they completed their educations. We were not aware of any of these fellows or scholars being trained in our Medical Center institutions. We were later disappointed to learn that one of the finest medical centers in the world, located in Howard Hughes's hometown, the city in which he and his father had been given the opportunity to make their start, was not to be a recipient of any of his accumulation of great wealth.[14]

Early in February, the president of the alumni association of the University of Kansas City College of Dentistry informed me that I had been selected to be the school's "Man of the Year." On March 8, a story appeared in the *Kansas City Times* announcing this award. It was heart warming to receive this award from the school where I had graduated from and where I had first taught.[15]

During the early months of 1954, two female scientists with the M. D. Anderson Hospital—Dr. Beatrix Cobb, a research and clinical psychologist, and Dr. Dorothy Cato, a psychiatrist who had worked in Galveston with Dr. Jack Ewalt—began a movement which was to develop into one of Texas' most aggressive forward steps. One day, the two called on me to discuss the need for a psychiatric research institute in the Medical Center. They had been active in other state movements to improve the methods of treating patients suffering from mental illness. Yet most of all they were interested in seeing a start made in Texas to prevent patients from becoming so seriously ill that it would be necessary to commit them to a state hospital. I assured them that the Medical Center was extremely interested in mental health and that the suggestion that they had made was one that should be pursued.

A short time later, on March 2, I received a letter from Governor Shivers asking me to serve as chairman of a special committee that would survey

Texas facilities for research and training in mental health. I gladly accepted the appointment. Later, I learned that Dr. Robert Sutherland of the Hogg Foundation at the University of Texas in Austin had suggested this action to the governor. Fourteen other prominent scientists and physicians were appointed as members of the committee. I was pleased to note that Dr. Eugene Kahn, professor of psychiatry at Baylor Medical School, and Dr. Laurie Calicutt, professor of psychology at the University of Houston, were to be on the committee. It was especially pleasing to me to learn that Dr. Beatrix Cobb also had been named as a member of the committee.

Soon after the committee was organized, we went to work. We were divided into groups to make surveys and studies of the various facilities that we were to visit. After several months of work, we prepared a detailed report that we presented to the governor. In it we reported our findings and made recommendations that we believed were necessary to correct the conditions that existed in the state hospitals. We also recommended a long-range plan for the development of teaching and research facilities for the state of Texas. All members of this committee could take pride in how many of our recommendations were carried out. Facilities for daycare treatment were established. State hospital facilities improved, and crowded conditions were relieved. Research programs in mental health were evident in institutions throughout the state. The creation of the Texas Research Institute of Mental Sciences, which was located in the Medical Center, was one of the major accomplishments. Throughout the state, many local mental health associations were established. These associations not only served to support the daycare facilities in their particular areas, but also to assist families and patients who were in need. If for nothing else, Governor Shivers should long be remembered by Texans for seeing to it that something was done to provide programs for treatment and research for one of the most widespread diseases of all, mental illness.

I should explain that the creation of this research institute was not as difficult as it might seem. At the last meeting of the committee, before submitting our report to the Governor, it was decided that a research institute was an immediate need. The committee asked me to determine how this might be done. With the help of the local members of the committee and Dr. William Lhamon, who had been appointed recently as chairman of the department of psychiatry at Baylor Medical School, we developed a plan for research and the treatment of patients. A building was planned that would provide laboratories for research and hospital facilities for the care of sixty patients.

When the plans were completed, I decided that I would discuss them with Vernon McGee, director of the Legislative Budget Board, and his assistant William Cobb, whom I knew well. I learned our committee's report had been in their hands for some time. The governor had requested them to study it. I informed McGee that I had brought with me preliminary plans for a research institute to be located in the Medical Center in Houston, and that I had prepared an outline of the functions that should be provided by this facility. I was pleased that they both agreed with our report to the governor. McGee stated bluntly that something had to be done to improve the unacceptable conditions existing in the state hospitals. He also said that a concerted effort should be made to provide a facility such as a psychiatric institute that might be successful in lowering the admission rate to the state hospitals. McGee as much as said that, "We want this research institute as of yesterday." I admired the efficiency with which McGee and Cobb approached this subject. They were well-informed in regard to the mental health conditions in the state. They also were concerned with the large appropriations that the legislature made each year to support the hospitals that they thought were providing inadequate care.

When I visited with Vernon McGee and William Cobb, the legislature was in session. I had arranged a meeting with the expectation that McGee might discuss the idea of researching mental disease with the legislators he was in constant contact with. I did not expect the surprising events that happened. Suddenly, William Cobb excused himself and left the room while I continued my discussion with Vernon McGee. I suggested to McGee that the institute could be located in the Medical Center as a unit of the University of Texas. Shortly, Cobb returned to the office and informed us that he had talked with the chairman of the House Appropriations Committee. The chairman wanted to know if it were possible for me to appear before his committee right away. This was a surprise, but I agreed to do so. Cobb said the chairman would have a page assist him in getting a quorum of the committee together. Cobb left, but in a short time he returned to tell me that the committee was assembled and that a quorum was present. I hurried with him to the meeting. The chairman introduced me to the members of the committee and explained that I had served as chairman of the Committee on Mental Health that had been appointed by Governor Shivers. He then asked me to report to the committee members our findings and our recommendations. I did so briefly. The chairman explained to the members of the committee that I had brought with me a preliminary plan for a psychiatric institute in the Texas Medical Center in Houston. Then he asked the committee, "Shall we provide for a state psychiatric institute at this session?" Approval was unanimous and Cobb was instructed to develop plans that the committee could approve. All this occurred in not more than an hour. I was astounded. I had no idea that this would occur when I planned my trip to Austin. Looking back at all of my previous appearances before committees while dean of the Dental Branch, I was amazed at this rapid action.

Later in March, another big day arrived for Lee Clark. The time had come to move about sixty patients from their beds in the framed army barracks buildings on Baldwin Street to their modern hospital beds in the beautifully decorated rooms of the new M. D. Anderson Cancer Hospital. It was a very satisfying day for all of us who remembered the beginning and an almost overwhelming one for Lee. This beautiful new building of pink marble inspired an editorial writer for the *Houston Chronicle* to take a long look at the Medical Center and then write, "There is no element of activity in this city which better exemplifies this spirit of Houston than the Texas Medical Center. Virtually every facet of the community's character is demonstrated in the pink marble building the great Medical Center just completed." [16]

It was proper, and to be expected of Lee, that on April 14, 1954, a portrait of Monroe D. Anderson, the man who had made the Medical Center and this hospital possible, was unveiled. Mayor Roy Hofheinz proclaimed Sunday, May 9, 1954, as "Medical Center Visitation Day." Members of the junior chamber of commerce were to serve as tour guides and police were present to control the traffic that was expected. It was a well-planned event, but rather a disappointment. Attendance was not as large as we had expected. This event was never repeated. In summing it up, we reasoned that the small turnout was due to the fact that, while Houstonians were most proud of their Medical Center, they did not wish to visit hospitals until it was absolutely necessary to do so.

In June, we moved our Medical Center offices from the Hermann Professional Building to the not quite finished Jesse H. Jones Library in the oval of the Medical Center. While the upper floor had been completed, some of the lower floors were in the final stages of construction. The passenger elevators were not operating so it was necessary to use the freight elevators. Our offices were located on the fourth floor. They were lovely. I had reduced the size of the planned space to about half of the area that Dr. Bertner had requested because it was not needed at that time. The Texas Medical Center offices would eventually occupy the quarters that were originally planned by Dr. Bertner.

On July 16, shortly after our move, the Doctor's Club had an opening party in their new quarters on the third floor of the library building. This was a happy occasion for the physicians who had spent many years looking forward to the day when they would have a library of their own. It was also a happy day for Dr. Claude Cody, Jr., and Dr. Moise Levy, who were largely responsible for obtaining the funds necessary to complete the building. With their wives in the receiving line, they greeted visitors as they arrived. At the time the doctors were hoping for such a building, they did not contemplate the added bonus of the Doctor's Club. It would be possible for various medical groups to arrange noon luncheons and evening dinner meetings for various functions. It was believed that this added convenience would induce members of the various medical groups to attend evening meetings.

One of the first visitors of note to the Medical Center was the Spanish dictator Generalissimmo Francisco Franco's only daughter, the Marquesa de Villaverde, and her husband, Dr. Christofo de Villaverde, a young chest surgeon. A visit by a countess to our Medical Center was not an everyday happening. They had been visiting many cities throughout the United States during the previous six weeks and on the last day of July they stopped in Houston for two or three days—the husband wished to visit the heart facilities that were here. As the years passed, we would have many visitors and patients of note to our Medical Center including kings, ex-kings, presidents, princesses, emperors, and more.[17]

Someday I should prepare a roster or list of names of the many people who helped develop and support the Texas Medical Center. Many people come to my mind. One of them, Dr. Paul V. Ledbetter, played an active part from the beginning, during the Texas Dental College days. He taught in the college without compensation, served on its board of trustees, and continued to teach in the School of Dentistry long after it had been moved to the Medical Center and after I had become director of the Medical Center. Dr. Ledbetter also devoted considerable energy to the Houston Heart Association during its early days. He brought many prominent doctors, such as Paul Dudley White, the physician for President Eisenhower during his critical days, to speak at meetings of physicians in Houston. In August, Dr. Ledbetter brought Dr. Isaac Berconsky of Buenos Aires to our city. Dr. Berconsky had performed the first heart catheterization. Dr. Ledbetter, a prominent Episcopalian, quietly served to help St. Luke's Hospital become a reality. This is but a small part of the background of one of the individuals that should be on the roster.

The latter part of August in Houston can be very warm and August 21, 1954, was such a day. Dr. Arthur Kirschbaum, who had recently been appointed professor of anatomy at the University of Texas M. D. Anderson Hospital, the Dental Branch, and at Baylor College of Medicine, was to arrive in Houston by plane with ten thousand mice. These precious lives made up a very valuable "germ-free" colony of mice. Dr. Kirschbaum had carefully bred this colony of mice for over seventeen years. If he lost his mice, he would have lost all these years. Kirschbaum had carefully planned his trip so that he would arrive in Houston early in the morning. His little mice could not live in temperatures above eighty degrees Fahrenheit. Things were moving smoothly until he and his entourage were blocked in traffic while still in Chicago. A fire caused the two hour delay. Fortunately, it was cold in Chicago, but the concern was arriving in Houston when it would be hot. They notified Dr. Stanley Olson of the unfortunate delay and he worked frantically to prepare for their arrival. He arranged for special air-conditioning equipment with large fans to blow cool air into the plane when it arrived. Also, air-conditioned vehicles were provided to carry the "visitors" to the Medical Center. A police escort even hurried the trip from the airport to the Medical Center and only forty-one mice died during the trip. Their deaths were due to cancer, the disease Dr. Kirschbaum was studying. These mice were the basis of his research. The M. D. Anderson Foundation provided a several thousand dollar grant to transport this colony of mice from Chicago to Houston. At the time, it was the only colony of its type in the world. This was a major event for the Medical Center.[18]

On September 10, after the transfer of books and other equipment from the other Medical Center libraries had been completed, the new Texas Medical Center Library in the Jesse H. Jones Building was dedicated. Many prominent citizens from Houston and elsewhere were present. Jesse H. Jones was presented a plaque in appreciation of the large grant that he had made for the construction of the building. Dr. Chauncey Leake, the vice president of the University of Texas Medical Branch, gave the principal address. During Dr. Leake's tenure as vice president of the Medical Branch, he had built a library that was considered one of the finest and most extensive medical libraries in the United States.[19]

The people of Houston, as they read their daily newspapers, may have thought that groundbreakings and dedications were daily occurrences in the Medical Center. It seemed that way, for on October 6, another dedication took place for St. Luke's Hospital even though patients were already in the hospital. Wright Morrow, president of the hospital's board of trustees, presided at the dedication ceremonies. Dr. Frank R. Bradley, president of the American Hospital Association, was the principal speaker, and Bishop Clinton S. Quin formally dedicated the hospital. It was to him that Mr. Cullen handed the $1 million dollar check to start the drive that brought this day to reality. After he had been introduced to the audience, Mr. Cullen remarked,

"I never dreamed that the 'small amount' of money that Lillie and I gave would turn out in such a big way."

Wright Morrow is one of the Medical Center greats whose name I must put on my list. He played an important part when he served as chairman of the fundraising committee for the chamber of commerce. This was during the time they were raising funds for the University of Texas at the Medical Center and the Baylor College of Medicine. He made several addresses throughout the years and his efforts required a considerable amount of his time.

The next great event to occur at the Medical Center was once again the dedication of a hospital. On October 23, 1954, Governor Shivers presided over the M. D. Anderson Hospital and Tumor Institute dedication. Many officials and friends were present to help dedicate a hospital that, in summation of the remarks made by the principal speaker, may well be the institution where the causes of the dreaded disease might be discovered. Among those the governor introduced were Arthur Cato, who, as a member of the House of Representatives, had introduced the bill for a cancer hospital during the 1941 session of the legislature. Then Governor Shivers introduced many prominent participants who were there, including Tom Sealy, chairman of the board of regents of the university; Dr. Logan Wilson, president of the university; U.S. Senator Price Daniel, who was Speaker of the House when Arthur Cato had introduced the bill that created the cancer hospital; County Judge Bob Casey; Mayor Roy Hofheinz; John Freeman, chairman of the board of the M. D. Anderson Foundation; and many others equally as prominent. Then he introduced Julia Bertner, the wife of E. W. Bertner who had died of the disease against which he had fought so hard. Julia knew Bill was smiling a proud smile that day.

About one month later, city officials proclaimed November 29, 1954, "Hugh Roy Cullen Day" in Houston. That day, Prentice-Hall Publishers released a book written by Ed Kilman and Theon Wright. Myron Boardman, vice president of Prentice-Hall, previously had made a special trip to Houston to convince Mr. Cullen that such a book should be written while he was still alive and kickin', as Mr. Cullen might have said. One little line in the book, a story that Mr. Cullen liked to repeat and tell with a chuckle, was about "the time I wrote a check on an Oklahoma bank for $5.00 and it bounced." His chuckle was in part due to the fact that he had written the check as a gift to the Salvation Army. "Hugh Roy Cullen Day" was a fitting close to a very busy 1954.[20]

As the new year began, the newsletter "Texas Medical Center News" started with the usual first-of-the-year "hopes and ambitions." Luther Rowsey, who was educated in journalism, served the Medical Center as a writer of feature stories that could be released to the press, giving the public news about what went on in the Medical Center that would not violate the code of ethics of the Harris County Medical Society. At the time, Luther was busy developing a news service publication for the institutions in the Medical Center. The pilot edition appeared on February 15, 1955. It was the first and last edition. This publication could have been an interesting and informative weekly for those connected with the institutions in the center. But, like so many of the projects we conceived that "died aborning," this project died because the underwriting funds were not available. It might have served as a stabilizing influence for the Medical Center institution staffs during a long-lasting controversy that was coming.

The controversy became a public issue that year. Quiet mutterings of concern actually had begun the day that plans for our Medical Center were announced—when headlines read that Baylor College of Medicine would be moved to Houston. There were quiet misgivings and then voiced concern about what might happen. Yet doubts and fears were allayed to a degree with explanations and reassurances from those who envisioned what the Medical Center would become. But as time passed, doubts and grumblings were expressed on each occasion that another institution was announced for the center. The new hospital was closer to becoming a reality, and a newspaper story predicting that it might actually be built that year could have been the reason for the more out-in-the-open controversy that was about to happen.

It was a year when many hopes and dreams were realized. Each day it seemed that some new technique or treatment was announced. Research had lifted the curtain a little higher to shed more light on some of the unknowns concerning disease. It was the year that the ravages of polio were brought to a halt by Dr. Salk. The Texas Medical Center had sped through the past days and years with alacrity. The press, the public, and the professions were becoming more interested in health matters. This alone was a good achievement if it was all the Medical Center did.

An editor of the *Houston Post* asked Dr. Chauncey Leake to tell the story about the early men in Texas medicine in the newspaper, and no one was more able to do this than Dr. Leake. He wrote, "One hundred years ago there were hardly enough people in Texas to pose a health problem." His full-page story was a revitalizing tonic that began the new year. His story closed on a heartwarming note: "The [Texas] Medical Center may indeed become one of the world's great achievements in medicine during the next century. It will be the intellectual contributions from the Center that will eventually establish its prestige and greatness." Just the night before this article appeared, the junior chamber of commerce had named Dr. Denton Cooley the city's "Outstanding Young Man." This was the type of intellectual achievement Dr. Leake spoke of.[21]

But open controversy began in March when it seemed that a city-county hospital in the Medical Center was a real possibility. Throughout the past year, many articles had appeared in the newspapers about the hospital—the headlines themselves told the story of what was going on. On July 22, 1948, the headline "500,000 Sought for TB Hospital" appeared (at first it was to be a tuberculosis hospital). The same day, another headline read, "Medical Center May Be Site of New TB Hospital." On November 3, 1948, another read, "J. D. Hospital, Baylor College of Medicine Join Hands." This really started the grumblings. Then, on December 23, 1948: "City to Build Hospital Next Year, Mayor Says." On and on the stories appeared. On July 20, 1949: "Jefferson Davis Under Plan to be TB Unit." Then the announcement was made that a new five million dollar general, and not tuberculosis, hospital was being planned for the Medical Center. County Judge Glenn Perry was quoted saying, "It is the best news I've heard. As I see it, the plan is an excellent idea—personally I'm all for it."

Then the next day another headline appeared: "Cullen Assures Hospital." Roy Cullen was quoted: "The entire future of the Medical Center depends on the city's participation." Announcements like these continued to appear through the years, from 1950 to 1954, yet still no hospital. During 1955, the headlines took a different turn and became both ominous and sad in tone: "Play Doctors for Opposing Hospital Plan." Another: "Stand By Doctors Against Hospital Unit Draws Fire." Yet another: "Leaders Rally Past to Support Hospital." Bitter words began to fly as the argument pitted doctor against doctor and citizen against citizen. It developed into a frenzy that, to me, was created by fear—the fear of humans for time eternal—fear for survival.

The hospital seemed to be a threat to some physicians. But only time would tell the story. The hospital district plan, which had been approved by the legislature in 1953, was at the heart of the controversy. The law, as passed, permitted cities or counties of one hundred thousand in population to establish a hospital district similar to that of a school district, provided that the voters of the city or county approved. The voters did not approve a hospital district for Houston and Harris County in the year 1955.

On Sunday, May 1, an article appeared in the *Houston Chronicle* that added a note of cheer in the midst of the controversy. A picture appeared, with an announcement that Jo Lynn Clark, Lee Clark's daughter, had been named an outstanding member of the Junior Achievement of Houston, and that she would be one of the two principal speakers at a dinner to be given at the Rice Hotel on May 12. For Jo Lynn, this was an achievement that far surpassed anything that Daddy had ever done.

From June until September, the bitterness that was expressed over the proposed city-county hospital became so intense that years would pass before enemies would become acquaintances again. Once the discussions became controversial, I remained silent. On June 29, I made my last public appearance to explain the many distinct advantages that the location of the hospital in the Medical Center would bring to the people of Houston and Harris County. Now it was no longer proper for me, as director of the Medical Center, to make comments, a position that was difficult to maintain with the chiding that I had to take from both opponents and proponents—all friends of mine.

During the heat of passion, the Postgraduate Medical Assembly of South Texas demonstrated that some physicians appreciated very much what the Medical Center meant to them. At a luncheon given by the assembly on July 18, 1955, for Colonel Bates and John Freeman, the assembly presented plaques to them for their "unselfish devotion to humanity and outstanding contributions to medicine and surgery." The announcement of these awards and the warmth of the article that told the story behind the awards no doubt pricked the consciences of some who had been making bitter comments about the center.

I appreciated the expression of friendship that I received on the night of November 30, when I was honored with a dinner given by the Houston District Dental Society. They surprised me by bringing to Houston two of my first students from the time that I had taught in Kansas City. Both had risen to positions of prominence in the dental profession. Dr. Ralph Edwards was a professor of the University of Kansas City School of Medicine and Dr. Fred Richmond was vice president of the American Dental Association.

In December, the public learned again that there would be another dedication in the Medical Center. On December 2, 1955, the University of Texas Dental Branch building was finally dedicated. Many outstanding dentists and citizens of Texas attended the ceremony. It was a proud day for Dr. John V. Olson, dean of the school, and his faculty. They had been through strenuous days to make this occasion possible. Dr. Paul Ledbetter, who served the dental school for so many years, made some brief remarks during this ceremony. He said, "Today we see dentistry as a member of a great medical team, not as a branch to be handled on the side." It was a happy and fitting occasion for the close of the year.[22]

Making History
The Growth of the Texas Medical Center, 1956–59

~

THE NEW YEAR BROUGHT a new proposal by Roy Cullen for solving the problem of medical school-hospital relations. On January 10, 1956, Cullen sent a long wire message to the leaders of both the United States House of Representatives and the Senate urging them to warn the nation's businessmen to make contributions to health and educational services. Cullen's view was that if private funds became more available, it would not be necessary to ask the taxpayers to support hospitals that were associated with a medical school. This was the principal objection of those opposing the construction of the city-county hospital in the Medical Center. It was to be associated with Baylor University Medical School. Of course, Cullen's plan was too practical for Congress to even consider.

Later on in January, we were pleased to note that an originator of new techniques in photographic art, Gene Davis, the quiet and unassuming medical photographer for Methodist Hospital, was given an award at an international exhibit of photographic techniques in Brussels. His excellent portrayal of surgical procedures by motion pictures was of noteworthy quality. His work exemplified the value of the projected picture in teaching and would record accounts that would someday make a valuable library collection.

Sometimes exciting and profound events occurred that opened entirely new fields of pursuit for scientists. On April 13, 1956, it was announced that Dr. Roger Guillemin and his associates had discovered a vital brain hormone. He found that the tiny anterior pituitary body, the producer of six or more known hormones, had, as a controlling agent, the hypothalamus. What would come from this valuable discovery still lay ahead, but it is one of the rewards that can be heaped on those who made the Medical Center possible. Without the facilities that were available at Baylor Medical School, where Dr. Guillemin served as a neuroendocrinologist and physiologist, his group would not have made such a discovery. Unfortunately, the Medical Center lost Dr. Guillemin when he accepted an appointment at another institution where he could be associated with many more scientists in the same field.[1]

Another refreshing event occurred on May 9, 1956, when the building for the Institute of Religion, the first in the United States located in a medical center, was dedicated. The institute was to serve as a training and research institute for ministers, physicians, and others. It was a major goal of the institute to train graduate theological students to serve more effectively as hospital chaplains.

Also in May, two other satisfactory events occurred. One was the $160,000 gift to Baylor Medical School by the Mading Foundation. This gift was given for the purpose of expanding the research and teaching facilities in surgery at the medical school. Gifts such as this were sparks that renewed the enthusiasm of all who served in the Medical Center. The other event was the announcement made by Methodist Hospital, in the latter part of May, that they must expand their facilities. This need marked the good that the hospital was accomplishing. The expansion program underway at Methodist Hospital presaged what was to happen in the Medical Center through the years—expansion after expansion, new buildings, and new programs.

In the latter part of June, another expansion was announced when Logan Wilson, president of the University of Texas, reported that the board of regents had approved an $800,000 request for expansion of the M. D. Anderson Hospital. The expansion would provide office facilities on the seventh floor of the building. This area had been an open deck, and it was to be enclosed and subdivided into offices for administration, which had been on the first floor. The first floor area, previously used for administration, would be used to expand badly needed clinical facilities. From the time the hospital opened, the clinic area had always been overcrowded and could not keep pace with the demands for its services. Patients came from far and wide because the hospital was becoming widely known throughout Texas and the United States.

In the latter part of June, Ross Garrett and his associates had completed the study that they had been making of hospital facilities in Houston and Harris County. Garrett also made his report to a joint meeting of the city council and the county commissioners. It was an informative and factual report. Following Garrett's explanation of the report, he was asked critical questions concerning the [city-county] hospital, which he recommended be built in the Medical Center. Commissioners wondered if Houston taxpayers would be subsidizing a private medical school. Garrett replied that,

based upon his study, they would not. Garrett mentioned that Baylor's participation in medical care at Jefferson Davis hospital was responsible for raising
the hospital's standards to the degree that residents and interns were being
attracted to it from medical schools throughout the United States. Then a
question from Councilman Louis Welch (later mayor of Houston), "Does
this increase in the number of doctors cause an increase in hospital costs?"
Garrett stated that his plan would decrease hospital costs. The discussion
took place in a public hearing that served to remove much of the public sus-
picion concerning the building of the hospital in the Medical Center, but
still did not alter the stand of many opponents.

In August, Dr. Leon Dmochowski received a ten thousand dollar grant
from the American Cancer Society to assist in the continuation of his study
of viruses as they related to cancer. Dr. Dmochowski was conducting this
research as part of a joint project of Baylor Medical College and the Anderson hospital. This research endeavor emphasizes the many years that scientists devoted to the search for a specific cause of a condition. Dr. Dmochowski had spent many years studying the relation of viruses to cancer, and his
findings were of significant importance. He never relaxed his pursuit. Dr.
Dmochowski later announced that he had isolated a virus that caused cancer in mice and said that it would reproduce cancer in other mice. This announcement caused scientists throughout the United States to renew their
interest in viruses as causative agents of some types of cancer.

Waning energies were often reinvigorated when praises were made of accomplishments. This was especially true for those of us at the Medical Center who read the September issue of *Houston Business*. This publication of
business achievements in Houston was published frequently by the chamber of commerce. The headline alone was stimulating: "Medical Center
Mirrors Houston's Growth." The issue was devoted almost entirely to the
Medical Center. There was an aerial view of the Medical Center, along with
pictures of the complete buildings illustrating the story. Naturally, we responded with a warm thanks to the editor.

On September 27, 1956, an enthusiastic visitor to our Medical Center
brought a glow of pride to those who had planned and built the Texas Children's Hospital. The wife of the vice president of the United States, Pat
Nixon, commented after her visit, "The finest I've ever seen." That statement alone was enough to swell the chest of Lep Meyer, who, along with
other officials of the hospital, toured the facility with her. All of us who had
the opportunity to meet Mrs. Nixon found her to be a charming lady.[2]

The future of the University of Texas Cancer Foundation was assured by a $100,000 grant from the Anderson Foundation made in November. This was to be an annual grant for five years, totaling $500,000. The worthiness of this grant, like all the other grants made by the trustees of the Anderson Foundation, has been demonstrated over time. The trustees of the M. D. Anderson Foundation have been lauded many times for their careful and expert management of the funds with which they had been entrusted.

Dr. Bertner would have been pleased with the news that the Gulf Coast Medical Foundation had been established in Wharton, Texas, the home of Mr. and Mrs. Marshall Johnson. Dr. Blasingame, one of the leading physicians in the Wharton community, played an active part in the organization of the foundation. The purpose of the foundation as stated in their public announcement, was "to improve the health of the people in this area." It was an early dream of the Texas Medical Center's to serve as a hub for hospitals and clinics located in the smaller communities, so that the Medical Center health team would be available for consultations with these local physicians. As the speaker for this occasion, I mentioned in my remarks that Dr. Bertner had emphasized this relationship early in the history of the Medical Center. Even though this particular dream of theirs did not develop to the degree that Dr. Blasingame had envisioned, the Texas Medical Center has continued through the years to be a source of new information for physicians throughout the surrounding area.

As the years passed, the eyes of not only Texas, but also of the world, were upon us. The first of a series of television broadcasts sponsored by the Ciba Corporation (a pharmaceutical manufacturing company), "Medical Horizons," was televised over the ABC network from the University of Texas Dental Branch on March 3, 1957. The broadcast was channeled through Houston's Channel 13 at 3:30 in the afternoon. The broadcast was followed by others that concerned health issues from the Mayo Clinic, Yale University, the University of California, the University of Pennsylvania, and other universities and hospitals throughout the United States. No doubt the Dental Branch was chosen as the first institution to broadcast from since it had become widely known for its complete television teaching facilities. Engineers from the Radio Corporation of America had assisted the architects in planning the television system when building plans for the dental school were being developed. This was a spectacular affair for the dental school. Mobile crews from Channel 13 moved in with sound trucks, sound engineers, and studio directors from ABC. Twenty-seven technicians, several engineers from Channel 13, and the technical director from ABC were there. Of course, the cast from the Dental Branch was there, too—six professors and their patients. The beginning of this series of broadcasts had been

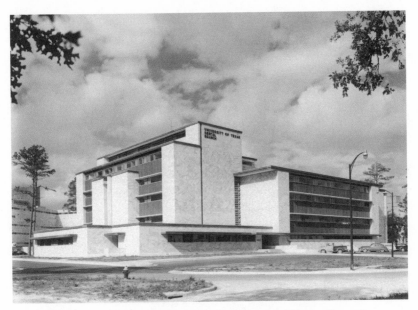

University of Texas Dental Branch, Texas Medical Center, circa 1955.

widely publicized by the press throughout the United States. This was yet another first for the Medical Center.[3]

In the latter part of December, 1956, the trustees of the Ford Foundation had announced that during the next year, $500 million would be distributed to various educational and medical institutions throughout the world. Ninety million dollars of this large distribution was to go to forty-five medical schools in the United States. On March 29, 1957, Baylor Medical School was notified that it would be the recipient of a two million dollar grant. We were all pleased that the stature of the Medical Center and Baylor had risen to the point that national foundations felt secure in making grants of such magnitude to our institutions.

Earlier I discussed my appearance before a committee of the Texas House of Representatives concerning a psychiatric institute. I had been surprised by the committee's quick acceptance and approval of this proposal. Now, on May 19, a news release from Austin carried the information that the bill that was prepared at the request of the committee chairman had passed the House unanimously. It had also passed the Senate with only one amendment added. The bill located the psychiatric institute in the Texas Medical Center in Houston. It was a happy announcement.

Helen Holt (later Garrott) had served for a long time as an untiring worker in the development of the library. For almost thirty years Helen had worked in facilities not planned for a library. First it was quarters in the medical arts building (a professional building for physicians and dentists), then it was in temporary quarters at Baylor Medical School in the Medical Center. Only during the last three or four years before her retirement did Helen have the pleasure of working in facilities that were actually planned for a medical library. Virginia Parker succeeded Helen as our new Medical librarian. She was a graduate of Newcomb College of Tulane University, and she had previously received a B.S. degree in library science. Through the years until my retirement, I had the pleasure of working with Miss Parker. The library offices on the first floor were convenient for me—just an elevator ride down from the fourth floor.

The manner in which the Medical Center had been established and was operated attracted many visitors who were interested in developing a similar plan for their centers. Almost all other medical centers in the United States were outgrowths of medical schools and were controlled by them. Ours was different: the medical schools here were related to the other institutions on a cooperative basis. Early in the year, I had two visitors call on me who were interested in a medical center for San Antonio. I was puzzled because they did not mention a relationship with any group in their city. I told them that if a group was interested in a medical center, I would be glad to visit San Antonio and discuss a plan with them. It was then that they told me that they were in real estate and had a very large tract of land that they wished to develop as a residential district with a medical center nearby. They inferred that they would donate a large tract of ground for medical center purposes. This was an interesting revelation. I informed them that a larger tract of ground would be needed for their medical center than what the Texas Medical Center had. I pointed out to them that we had outgrown our original tract of 134 acres within just twelve years. I also mentioned that to plan a medical center without providing for an outlying area where less expensive land could be procured for parking would be a serious mistake. I showed them the model of the monorail system that was prepared by the planning engineers at the Medical Center. Although our monorail system plan was dead, I stressed the wonderful opportunity that they had to include a monorail system in their own plans. With the amount of land that they had available for development, I suggested it would be possible to develop a large residential area nearby for those who wished to retire in San Antonio. They also could include a business district in their plans that would be near the medical center and residential areas that could be served by the monorail system. This would give the residents, faculty, students, and others the opportunity to travel from one area to another without an automobile, thus reducing automobile traffic in the medical center. It was a visionary dream of mine, yet it seemed to me to be a plausible and practical one. One of the visitors remarked, "I'm afraid this idea is too far out in front for us." I had heard this type of remark before.

Dr. James Hollers, a prominent dentist and president of the San Antonio Medical Foundation, contacted me in the latter part of May. He asked if I would be available for a trip to San Antonio to discuss with the trustees of the medical foundation the possibility of a medical center for San Antonio. Naturally, I presumed that this was the outcome of the earlier conversation that I had with the two gentlemen from San Antonio. Years later, I learned that this was not the case. Dr. Hollers was quite surprised to learn of their visit. He conjectured that their visit was to determine whether they should make a gift of land for this purpose. The trustees of the foundation had re-quested a tract from these developers earlier in the year. I made several trips to San Antonio to discuss the possibility of a center. First, I met with the San Antonio Medical Foundation and explained to them in detail the manner in which our Medical Center had been planned. I used charts and booklets, which I developed for this purpose. When I returned to Houston I drafted a detailed organizational plan for the medical center in San Antonio.

During the year, I addressed a public meeting of the chamber of com-merce, the members of Bexar County Medical Society, and other lay groups in San Antonio. I did this at no cost. Other administrators from our Medi-cal Center institutions visited cities and addressed groups that were inter-ested in us and our plan of operation. Thanks to the untiring efforts of Dr. James Hollers, the South Texas Medical Center came into being. It was mag-nificent center located on a beautiful tract of ground, with uncrowded facil-ities, and beautified with trees, flowers, and shrubbery. In a short time, a University of Texas health center, which included a medical school, a nurs-ing school, a dental school, and other auxiliary educational facilities, was lo-cated in their city. Also a thousand-bed Veterans Administration Hospital, as well as a large Methodist Hospital, and several other medically-related en-terprises were located there.

Well-planned facilities for private medical activity surrounded the center. They included shops, a surgical supply store, and a medical bookstore. An attractive residential area was located nearby. The two gentlemen who had visited me in Houston earlier had given two hundred acres of land to the trustees of the South Texas Medical Center. We, in our Medical Center, felt quite pleased with the important role that we played in assisting the people of San Antonio to develop an outstanding medical center for the state of Texas and the United States. Sadly, only a short time after the last time I visited Dr. Hollers, his death was announced in the San Antonio newspapers. I quote from one: "Flags are flying at half-mast over the Audie Murphy Veterans Hospital and more than twenty institutions in the South Texas Medical Center—Jim Hollers has passed on. His work will live on. Our city, state, and nation will miss him." I add, "Indeed they will."

From the start, it was determined that some means of controlling the coordination of relationships between the various institutions in the Medical Center should be included in the restrictions that were made a part of the deed. It was not the intention of the Medical Center's board of trustees to interfere with the internal organization and operations of the individual institutions. We used the expression "horizontal cooperation—vertical operation." Restrictions that were prepared required each institution to meet certain standards and to cooperate in certain activities such as providing teaching beds for use of the teaching institutions—a requirement for all of the hospitals. Other similar restrictions were made a part of the deed, but no policing method was included. We knew that the good will of the institutions was all that would be required and it was. Earlier, competition between some institutions seemed to have been a motivating factor in the development of high quality research and high quality teaching in our Medical Center. Yet, I came to the conclusion that a stronger, centralized relationship would be to the advantage of all the institutions in the Texas Medical Center. I had in mind a relationship that would not interfere with the operation of each institution, but one that would provide for central control of the cooperative enterprises. I knew that if the plan I developed was adopted, changes might need to be made, depending upon the degree of resistance to the proposal. The plan would require the full cooperation of each Medical Center institution's board of trustees and also the cooperation of the trustees of all large foundations that were the principal supporters of the Medical Center. Months went into developing the plan. It was complicated to a degree because of the many diverse groups involved. Briefly, the plan included:

1. The board of trustees from each institution would be asked to appoint a medical representative.
2. Subject to approval by the Texas Medical Center board, representatives from each institution were to serve as members of the Medical Center Board of Governors.

3. The administrative officer of the Texas Medical Center would serve as overseer.
4. The Texas Medical Center board would approve all policy matters of the board of governors and the administrators.
5. The administrator of each institution would continue to be in complete charge of the institution, under the institution's board. All action of the board of governors, as the controlling authority for coordination, would be administered according to the policy of each institution.

It was a workable proposal, patterned after the operational plan of the Humble Oil and Refining Company. Hines Baker had loaned their organizational plan to me. In June, before it became known to others, I took the final draft of the plan to James Anderson, president of the Medical Center's board of trustees. However, the idea went no further and I dropped it as I had done with so many others. The Medical Center seems to have gotten along well without it.

On June 6, Methodist Hospital's $7.5 million plan for expansion was approved. At the Texas Annual Conference of the Methodist Church, O'Banion Williams, president of the hospital board, informed those attending the conference that they had approved the expansion plan. Also, the Medical Center's board of directors had approved the hospital's proposal for the establishment of an ongoing foundation structure that would be able to plan for future needs. The foundation structure that Williams announced in 1957 served Methodist Hospital well through the years. Facilities at the hospital eventually doubled in size from those that were available when the foundation plan was announced.

The city-county hospital controversy continued throughout 1957 as it had during the past several years. It was now becoming an almost routine activity, as far as discussions or arguments were concerned. Plan after plan was prepared by opposing groups to offset the plan of Baylor Medical School to be in control of the medical staff of the hospital. The situation continued to be a headache for city and county officials alike. They felt it was their responsibility to settle the matter so that they could do what the taxpayers had authorized them to do—to build a new hospital so that care of the indigent could be improved. Yet the members of the two groups, the city council and the county commissioners, were continually confused by the various plans which were being proposed. It had become almost a weekly occurrence for them to hold meetings to discuss the hospital issue. After these meetings, their comments to the press illustrated their confusion. City councilman George Kessler remarked, "I'm for any practical plan that the Medical Society or anyone else can come up with to improve Jefferson Davis Hospital. However, such a program as recommended by the Medical Society would be unworkable. It is as though each member of the City Council has authority to tell the various department heads what to do." The Medical Society had recommended that the staffing of the hospital should be done by three different groups. Then a sidestep reply made by another councilman: "I'm for anything that can be done to improve the quality of the medical care of the indigent sick of Houston and Harris County." Still no hospital in 1957.

Lamar Fleming, Jr., president of the Texas Institute for Rehabilitation and Research, announced on July 9 that sufficient funds were available to build a hospital for the institute, which had been operating in temporary facilities provided by the Wolf Home. The new building would be constructed on part of a tract of ground that had been deeded originally to Baylor University College of Medicine by the Anderson Foundation. Baylor had in turn given the tract for this building to the board of trustees of the rehabilitation institute. Bids for the building were to be called on August 15. The Knutson Construction Company submitted the low bid. Knutson's interest in children had long been demonstrated at the Shrine Crippled Children's Clinic where he supported many of their activities. During the construction of the building for the rehabilitation institute, the staff recommended many changes that they felt needed to be made. Knutson, who had quietly contributed to the construction of the building, made several of these changes without adding to the cost of the construction.

In September, the officers of the Good Samaritan Club announced plans to create a seven million dollar building for a nursing school in the Texas Medical Center at a banquet at the Rice Hotel. Not only was the building to provide quarters for the school of nursing, but also for large lecture rooms and a large auditorium. The plans also included facilities for several cafeterias and dining rooms. The banquet room at the Rice Hotel was filled. Bob Smith, an enthusiastic supporter of the project, presided. Dr. Charles Allen, a minister from Atlanta, Georgia gave the principal address. Dr. Allen would later become pastor of the First United Methodist Church in downtown Houston. This, however, became another project that died "aborning."

One of the last events of 1957 was the announcement of public support for the University of Texas Postgraduate Medical School. Dr. Grant Taylor, the dean, was at long last, after a determined and dogged effort, able to gain support for the school from the public. But, the legislature again passed the buck back to the Anderson Foundation and to the physicians who paid fees to attend courses given by the school. The regents of the University of Texas were determined not to let it go down the drain. Persistence and patience were rewarded. The postgraduate school became something more than had even been planned. It became the University of Texas Graduate School of Biomedical Sciences. Included in its program was a school for continuing education, which offered postgraduate courses to physicians, dentists, and the allied professions.

One of the first public reports in the new year of 1958 concerned the county morgue. Due largely to the efforts of Dr. William Russell, chief pathologist at M. D. Anderson Hospital, a specialist in forensic pathology had been appointed to become chief pathologist in the county medical examiner's office. The county medical examiner at the time was an outstanding Houston surgeon, Dr. Edward Clark. Dr. Clark had agreed to serve in this position for a short time while a reorganized program could be developed. With Dr. Russell's help, Dr. Clark obtained the services of Dr. Joseph A. Jachimczyk. Dr. Jachimczyk had been persuaded to come to Houston to accept the position. Within a short time the county commissioners knew that they had made a wise decision. Services were decidedly improved in the county medical examiner's office after Dr. Jachimczyk's arrival. Dr. Jachimczyk became recognized throughout the state of Texas. He made many contributions to various law agencies throughout the state, as well as contributed considerable information concerning infectious diseases to health departments and medical schools. He continued to serve many years in this position, and was even called upon to determine the cause of death of Howard Hughes.

It was to be another year of city-county hospital wrangling in 1958. It was headlined in a newspaper: "Cold War between City and County Stymies Work for More Facilities." The argument between the city and county officials was based primarily on who would operate and support the hospital— the city or the county. We continued to wait. Baylor's medical staff continued to serve Houston's indigent sick at Jefferson Davis Hospital, which, through the years of Houston's growth, had become totally inadequate for the care of patients in addition to serving as a teaching hospital.

In February, the Medical Center allocated a tract of ground to the state hospital board as a site for the new State Psychiatric Institute for Mental Research. The site allocated was near Baylor College of Medicine so that the psychiatric staff of the medical school could serve the institute better. Sixty beds would be available when the institute was completed. In May, Dr. Cyril J.

Ruilman, Tennessee's Commissioner of Mental Health, was appointed director of the Texas Hospital System. The chairman of the hospital board, Howard Tellepson, asked me to assist in the board's selection of the hospital director. I talked with Dr. Hyman, vice president of the University of Tennessee Medical Center in Memphis, concerning Dr. Ruilman. Dr. Ruilman was serving also as a professor of mental health at the University of Tennessee Medical Center. Dr. Hyman highly recommended Dr. Ruilman. Previously, plans were made to use the old facilities of the M. D. Anderson Hospital on Baldwin Street as temporary quarters for the psychiatric institute. Some confusion developed over this arrangement because of a misunderstanding at Jefferson Davis Hospital. It had been presumed by the maternity ward staff at Jefferson Davis hospital that the old cancer hospital facilities were to be used as a temporary facility for maternity patients. The difficulty was resolved when the hospital board announced that temporary quarters for maternity cases would be provided on a site to the rear of Jefferson Davis Hospital, a much more satisfactory arrangement for the staff and for the patients.

In February, the first noise pollution meeting was held in the Texas Medical Center library auditorium. The meeting was arranged by the Texas Medical Center, the Speech and Hearing Center, and the Gulf Coast Section of the American Industrial Hygiene Association. The main theme of the meeting was a discussion of industrial noise as a health menace. The rapid increase of industry in the Houston area had prompted the Industrial Hygiene Association to hold their meeting at our Medical Center.

In the latter part of February, I was asked by the Amarillo Chamber of Commerce to speak to the city's various medical and civic groups concerning a medical center for their city. At the time it seemed to me that their program should be directed more toward an ancillary medical education program rather than to attempt a program in medical and dental education. I felt that the legislature probably would not consider other medical and dental schools in Texas during the time that they were considering a medical school in San Antonio. I was wrong. A medical school was established later in Lubbock, and Amarillo developed an excellent medical center for comprehensive medical care.

Often overlooked was the fine work done by business enterprises. Not only did they continue to make annual grants to various educational and medical research institutions, but they also planned events that would benefit some worthwhile projects. One of Houston's leading stores, Sakowitz, planned a fashion extravaganza in April for the benefit of the eye institute in the Medical Center. The Eyes of Texas Foundation had been chartered by the state as a charitable foundation for the prevention of blindness through education, teaching, and research. The Eyes of Texas Foundation was the beneficiary of the Sakowitz extravaganza. The "Summer is a Song" event was presented in the Emerald Room of the Shamrock Hotel and had over one thousand guests. Ray Elliott, of Sakowitz Brothers, was largely responsible for the success of the event. Later, the Lions Club banded together with the three television stations in Houston and sponsored a giant telethon. Ray Elliott was chairman of the committee that directed the telethon, which began on a Saturday at 11 P.M., and ended on Sunday at 5 P.M. Donors contributed $56,000 for the construction of the eye institue building in the Texas Medical Center. Dr. Louis Girard served as director of the institute, which was later located in the Jewish Research Institute building.

In May of 1958, we were saddened by the death of Dr. Arthur Kirschbaum. Dr. Kirschbaum had brought the mouse colony from Chicago. He was only forty-seven years old. A coronary snuffed out the life of one who had devoted his research to saving other lives. Those who were engaged in heart disease research, both in the laboratories and in the hospitals, were quite distressed over the loss of one of their coworkers.[4]

Back in March, 1952, the first cobalt unit for cancer treatment was installed in the cancer hospital. Now, in July, 1958, it was announced that an entirely new unit would take the place of the first one, which had been a cooperative development of Drs. Fletcher and Grimmett. The new unit, likewise, was developed at the cancer hospital by Dr. Gilbert Fletcher and Dr. W. K. Sinclair, in cooperation with General Electric engineers and the Atomic Energy Commission of Canada. This new unit was twice as powerful as the first unit. Also the control mechanism was developed to the degree that the cobalt beam could be confined to an area of not more than 1/1000 of an inch. Research projects like this could make rapid progress when situated in quarters suitable for their purpose.

It was only a few days after the announcement was made about the new cobalt unit that James E. Anderson died. It was a sad loss for all of us in the Medical Center who knew Anderson well and had the pleasure of working with him at the cancer hospital. His devoted counsel, advice, and the contacts that he made accounted for the success of many of the programs inaugurated at the cancer hospital. He and Lee Clark were warm friends and worked closely together. Dr. Clark valued his counsel and advice. One of Anderson's noteworthy achievements was his effort towards establishing the University of Texas Cancer Foundation, serving as its first president. James Anderson died of cancer in the very hospital that was named after his uncle,

Monroe Dunaway Anderson. His father and uncles were the founders of the huge cotton company Anderson, Clayton & Company, a worldwide organization. Two of his brothers, Tom (who followed James as president of the Cancer Foundation) and Leland, continued to work in the Medical Center. Leland Anderson served as president of the Texas Medical Center after Dr. Bertner's death.[5]

Another first for our Medical Center began July 24, when our heliport, the first of its type in Houston, was opened. Great hopes were held for the success of this venture operated by Airlift, Inc. The Texas Medical Center board had received a small grant for the construction of the heliport and provided the funds for the fence and landing pad, which was located south of St. Luke's Hospital. It was dedicated by Mayor Louis Cutrer, who was the "first patient" to arrive in the ambulance helicopter at the heliport. David Saville, an executive of Airlift, accompanied him. Leland Anderson, the Medical Center president, and the administrators of our hospitals were present to greet the mayor as he stepped from the helicopter. Anderson, in a few brief remarks, explained the purpose of this new type of ambulance service. Emergency patients traveling by plane would be transferred from the airport to the Medical Center. Likewise, victims of industrial accidents or highway accidents could be picked up at the site of the accident and brought to the Medical Center in the helicopter in a short time. This, Anderson explained, was expected to save many lives. This was another idea, though actually underway, that died "aborning." No one called for the service during its entire operation. Only one patient was brought to the center by the helicopter ambulance, and the company ceased to exist.[6]

The last day of July served as another groundbreaking day, this time for the Speech and Hearing Center. At long last Dr. Charles Dickson was able to see one of his pet projects underway in its own building. He had been instrumental in beginning the project and in encouraging its development in the basement of Methodist Hospital. A committee headed by J. S. Cullinan II had raised funds for construction of the building. Other members of his committee included Dr. Dickson, Dr. Herbert Harris, and Gus Wortham. Cullinan's father, many years previous, had provided funds for the construction of the Houston Negro Hospital. Several years before, I had served on many Houston civic committees with his sister, Nina Cullinan. Miss Cullinan was a patron of the arts for many years. Houston people really were something else.

In August, Gene Wilburn, medical writer for the *Houston Chronicle,* visited me almost daily seeking stories for publication. On one very hot day, Gene called upon me and his very first words when he saw me were, "What are you going to do about this traffic and parking situation?" This question prompted a story that he wrote called "Medical Center Traffic Headed for Big Jam." Neither Gene or I could have anticipated the big jam that would eventually occur. We had appointed a traffic committee of the council of administrators to study and make suggestions for means to control the problem. As a private enterprise, the Medical Center could not be provided with Houston police service. Traffic violators in the center could only be asked "please don't." This was not a very effective method. It was some time later that the committee reluctantly admitted that the Medical Center grounds must be closed to outsiders. Patients, their families, and the doctors had to have first privileges for parking, and a parking system was devised at that time. A satisfactory solution would have been the monorail system, which had been planned previously, but was too farfetched for the Medical Center Board of Trustees at the time.

When the Medical Center was first organized, a school of nursing was included in the plans, and the University of Houston was asked to consider establishing a school of nursing in the Medical Center. Colonel W. B. Bates had made the suggestion to Dr. Bertner and had asked him to talk with the officials of the university. Once it was done, it resulted in the opening of the School of Nursing of the University of Houston, which I mentioned earlier. When the University of Houston closed its school, the Medical Center requested that the University of Texas establish a School of Nursing in the Medical Center. Many meetings were held with university officials concerning a nursing school, but it became evident that they were reluctant to establish one. This, no doubt, was due to the operation of a school of nursing at the Medical Branch in Galveston.

Dr. Melvin A. Casberg, who had been vice president for medical affairs of the University of Texas since 1956, made many trips to Houston to meet with members of our board about the nursing school. He held many meetings with officials in Austin and at the Medical Branch in Galveston. His efforts were not successful. He had been appointed vice president for medical affairs to develop a coordinated medical program for all of the units of the university. His efforts through the years proved to be futile. It seemed that the failure of his efforts to develop a unified program of nursing education in our Medical Center was the last straw. He resigned his position as vice president of the university on August 31.

About a week later, Leroy Jeffers, a member of the board of regents of the University of Texas, called me by telephone to inform me that the university board of regents had decided that they would create a school of nursing in the Medical Center provided that we would deed a tract of ground for this purpose. Also, the Medical Center would be requested to build the buildings. It was evident from the manner in which Jeffers related this information to me that he was not in accord with the board's action. Jeffers had expressed his own hopes for a University of Texas School of Nursing in the Medical Center. After he told me this, I paused for a moment and then asked who would provide the funds for the operation of the school. This, he replied, would be the responsibility of the Medical Center. At a specially called meeting of the executive committee of the Medical Center, I related my conversation with Leroy Jeffers. It only took the executive committee a few minutes to decide not to accept the university's offer. Later, the Texas Medical Center Board of Trustees approved the action of the executive committee. At the meeting of the executive committee, John Jones, a member of the committee, mentioned that Texas Woman's University might be interested in the operation of a nursing school in our center. At the time, they were operating a nursing school in Dallas in conjunction with the Southwestern Medical School of the University of Texas. This suggestion was received with enthusiasm. I was instructed to contact Dr. John Guinn, president of Texas Woman's University, in Denton. It was only a day or two later that Dr. Guinn arrived at my office. Events happened rapidly. Dr. Guinn was an administrator of action. His board, other state agencies involved, and the attorney general all approved the plan within a short time.

On October 7, a full-page headline story in the *Houston Chronicle* announced that, "Texas Woman's University would operate a college of nursing in the Texas Medical Center." A story in the *Houston Post* the next day quoted me as saying, "The green light for go was the attorney general's ruling Tuesday, when he ruled that the approval for establishing this school by the Texas Commission of Higher Education was not required." At long last the Medical Center was to have a college of nursing operated by a State university. John Jones's suggestion developed into a monumental thing. Texas Woman's University expanded their facilities by adding an additional building in the Medical Center. All phases of nursing education were included in their education program, as well as other auxiliary educational programs that served in a team approach for treatment of the sick.

Finally for the year 1958, Rex Baker, a prominent Houston attorney, released the report of the University of Texas' special "Committee of 75." Baker, chairman of the committee, was Hines Baker's brother. The board of regents received the report on December 6. It was lengthy and consisted of an analysis of the University of Texas medical and dental operations. The report was factual, therefore it revealed many of the discrepancies that existed

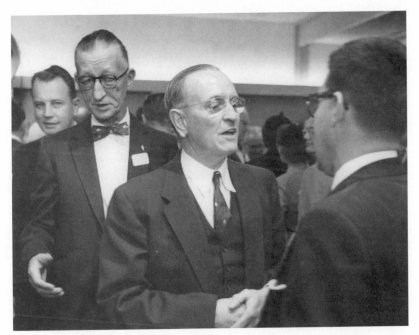

Elliott "working the crowd" in the mid-1950s. Courtesy E. W. D'Anton

in the various institutions. I felt that it was a helpful report in that it stimu-
lated the legislature and the people of Texas to take action for improving
their existing institutions that engaged in medical education. Also I believe
that it was helpful in many other areas of education on the main campus of
the university.

If any one year of the life of the Medical Center could be designated as
the most happy one, it should be the year of 1959. It seemed that 1959 was
the year that would forecast what was to occur in the Medical Center in the
years to follow. Those had who believed that their large gifts to the Medical
Center were sound investments could look to this year as ample proof of
their judgement. In every field of endeavor planned for the Medical Center—research, education, and patient care—report after report that year
more than justified the soundness of the Medical Center plan.

When it was finally announced that the Texas Woman's University would
build a College of Nursing in the Medical Center, the Good Samaritans'
board of trustees decided to develop a different much-needed facility for the
Medical Center. I had previously had many conversations with Clyde Verheyden, director of the Good Samaritans, concerning other programs—

some of which he had included in the nursing school building. We discussed with Bob Smith and other members of the Good Samaritan board, the idea of a commons building in the Medical Center. I mentioned to Verheyden that I had included this type of building in my annual report to the Medical Center Board. It would be an overall program that embraced several areas, such as health activities for the students and faculty (gym, tennis, bowling, swimming, and so forth). Second, it would have a large auditorium and smaller meeting rooms for organized society meetings. It would also include a small infirmary for students, a large cafeteria for the public, eating facilities for faculty and students, a guest dining room, and private dining rooms for dinner meetings. The building would provide space facing Fannin Street for a bookstore, a pharmacy, an orthopedic and surgical supply store, and other Medical Center-related enterprises. Office space would be provided for the Medical Center offices, as well as offices for all the allied health organizations.

A single building plan for all of these was a good thing at that time because ground space was in short supply. The building would occupy a 5.6-acre tract of ground. A large parking garage, below and above ground, was planned. In the beginning, the building would consist of thirteen floors and six wings. Each wing would serve different functions, planned around a traffic flow pattern that would facilitate easy access to all other related activities. Verheyden discussed the plan with his architects. They developed a magnificent structure that included a foundation that would support seven additional floors. Like so many of our other visionary ideas, the plan was dropped. Little enthusiasm could be aroused among our board members.

It would have been a self-supporting project operated by the Good Samaritans, but the board doubted that the plan would support itself. However, as Dr. Chauncey Leake explained to me later, a similar facility operated on University of California's medical campus and it was self-supporting. However, many felt that twelve million dollars for a building that would not be used for teaching and research was too much. The commons bulding was only one of six dreams that I suggested in my first-of-the-year report to the board of trustees. I also recommended the Institute of Life Chemistry; the Institute of Medical Literature and History (Dr. Chauncey Leake, director); the Distinguished Professor's Program (a "green pastures" idea); an endowment fund plan for the support of individual chairs in the teaching institutions; and, finally, an expanded library facility. Only one of my suggested programs was completed—the expanded library facility.[7]

In the middle of January, 1959, it was announced that Leon Jaworski had been appointed as chairman of the Joint Administrative Committee of the Texas Medical Center and Baylor University College of Medicine. Other members of the committee were John T. Jones, William A. Kirkland, John H. Freeman, Earl C. Hankamer, J. Sayles Leach, and George M. Irving. I served as secretary of the committee. It was announced that the committee would "deal with matters of policy and administration of the College of Medicine. It has already undertaken direction of the expansion program of the college which includes three new units." The organization came about primarily so that a closer working relationship could be developed for the construction of the college's three new buildings, which were badly needed.

Dr. Stanley Olson, dean of the medical school, had learned that the Department of Health, Education and Welfare might make a large grant available if it could be matched by funds provided by the Medical College. The administrative policy of the parent university in Waco did not permit the college of medicine to seek a grant from Washington. Succinctly stated, funds from Washington were "verboten." The Medical Center Board of Trustees, upon request of the Baylor College of Medicine, agreed to assume the responsibility for building. Grants to match the one obtained from the Department of Health, Education and Welfare for construction of the building were made by Houston Endowment, the M. D. Anderson Foundation, and the Jewish community of Houston. Later, Mr. and Mrs. Newton Rayzor provided funds for a connecting building. The gifts were ample. The Medical Center Board of Trustees made the request for the Department of Health, Education and Welfare grant. In due time the grant was approved and funds were made available for the construction of a building. All construction plans and supervision for the building were under the direction of the Joint Administrative Committee. Dean Stanley Olson and his faculty had planned the building and were responsible for recommending change orders if and when they were needed. Thus the Jesse H. Jones building, the M. D. Anderson building, the Newton Rayzor building, and the Jewish Research Institute building for the medical school were made possible by this arrangement. Leon Jaworski, in his usual manner of thoroughness, devoted considerable time and energy to his chairmanship of the Joint Administrative Committee. It was largely through his efforts that other members of the committee gave considerable time to the construction of the building. Later, this Joint Administrative Committee was disbanded.

On the first of February, one of my dreams appeared in the paper. The headline read: "Multimillion Tunnell Planned." Very early on, the way that people could travel from one building to the other in the Medical Center had been discussed. It was sometime in 1946 or 1947 that meetings were held with R. Kenneth Franzheim and his engineers concerning a tunnel system. Dr. Bertner and I had suggested a tunnel similar to the one at the Mayo Clinic. Franzheim was requested to conduct a feasibility study of this plan. He reported to the board that the idea would be a costly venture and that water barricades would need to be constructed. The idea was dropped.

In the latter part of 1959, we discussed again a tunnel connecting the medical school and Texas Woman's University, since the students of Texas Woman's University would be attending classes at the medical school. A tunnel was planned that would connect the Texas Woman's University to the Good Samaritan building when it was completed. Then another tunnel could be constructed that would connect the Good Samaritan building with the Methodist Hospital and St. Luke's Hospital. Engineers who made the preliminary study informed us that the cost, estimated to be about two hundred dollars a running foot, would be prohibitive. At the time I released the story to Gene Wilburn at the *Houston Chronicle,* this idea had not yet been dropped.

On March 12, 1959, at a dinner sponsored by the Texas Medical Center in celebration of its fifteenth anniversary, an announcement was made concerning the funds that had been given to the Texas Medical Center for the medical school buildings. A series of colored slides were shown of the buildings to be constructed. The story that appeared in the newspaper stated, "$25 million in buildings were planned which would be added to the $80 million already constructed." Some of the speakers congratulated the scientists from Baylor University College of Medicine for the many contributions they had made in research during the years. Likewise expressions were made that held high hopes for the Medical Center in the years to come. Oveta Culp Hobby, former member of the Medical Center Board of Trustees, who was then serving as Secretary of Health, Education, and Welfare in Washington, sent a wire to the board. "The health problem of the nation," she wrote, "should and can be solved by voluntary effort under the system of American Private Enterprise. American industries' acceptance of a share of the responsibility for aiding United States medical education so far has been heartening. It holds real promise for the future." Us oldtimers felt a warm glow as we left for home that evening.[8]

On March 6, there was a new arrival at the M. D. Anderson Hospital and Tumor Institute. A Cesium-17 unit was put into operation to be used primarily in the fight against breast cancer. It was hoped that the Cesium-17 unit would be so successful that radical type surgery could be eliminated.

Sadly, this was not been the case. Hope after hope was dashed to the ground by this destroyer of lives, cancer.

Early in the year, two people associated with the Medical Center died. One of them was Kenneth Franzheim, a well-known Houston architect. On March 19, 1959, it was announced that he had put in trust a fund for medical research and for a medical museum. Franzheim was one of Dr. Bertner's close friends, and he was the first architect to plan a building in the Medical Center—the Baylor University College of Medicine. On April 2, one of our early leaders, Dr. Walter Moursund, died. Dr. Moursund had served as dean of Baylor University College of Medicine for over thirty years, probably longer than any other medical school dean in the United States. During his tenure, he had been subjected to the trials and tribulations that often confront a dean, including war and confrontation after confrontation with medical groups. He managed this so well that he lost very few medical friends. Later he was to move a certain medical school from Dallas to Houston with such dispatch that the school continued its program of education without interruption. The board of trustees named a street after Moursund. Many of us were surprised when Dr. Stanley Olson was mentioned as a top candidate for the presidency at Baylor University in Waco. This was on the morning after the announcement of Dr. Moursund's death. Dr. Olson refused to comment since he was somewhat surprised that he was being considered. However, Dr. Olson continued as dean of the medical school and was not appointed president of the main university.[9]

On April 4, 1959, the story was out. A newspaper headline read: "Two Give $7 Million to Build Hospital. Identity of Couple Secret." The story continued to tell that the gift, possibly the largest such gift in Houston history, was given to the Lutheran Hospital Association for the construction of a 250-bed hospital in the Texas Medical Center.[10]

On April 12, Gene Wilburn again published one of his daily visits with me at the Medical Center in the newspaper. Headlines read: "Plan Medical Expansion Skyward." Gene made some of my dreams sound real. He listed some of my ideas.

The program as outlined includes:
1. The world's first Institute of Life Chemistry
2. At least four large parking garages
3. A Public Health College
4. An Institute of Geriatrics
5. Expansion of graduate education programs

The story went on to quote that "$48.5 million in buildings were approved for construction. This would bring the value of Medical Center buildings to $110 million." Gene had included the twelve million dollars that had been announced as the cost for the Good Samaritan building. It seems that my conversations must have inspired Gene about the possibility for an Institute of Life Chemistry. He wrote this part of his story as an appeal to philanthropists to support the project. While his story was dramatic, and in press jargon, it did make the wires.

Dr. James A. Green, the oldest member of the Baylor University College of Medicine faculty announced that he would retire from teaching and enter private practice. He was the longtime professor of medicine, and his joviality and warmth would be missed by the students. His chair was to be occupied by Dr. Raymond D. Pruitt, who, at the time of his appointment, was on the staff of the Mayo Clinic in Rochester and a member of the graduate faculty of the University of Minnesota School of Medicine. His appointment was announced on May 4, 1959.

Earlier, I mentioned briefly that I would be honored as "Dentist of the Century." I received this award on May 17, 1959. The award was made by the Houston District Dental Society as a part of the American Dental Association's celebration of its founding one hundred years earlier. The officers of the dental society had invited James Robinson, who represented the American Dental Association, to make the principal address. Robinson was a longtime friend of mine. He confined his remarks to events that had occurred in American dentistry during the preceding one hundred years. I have regarded this award as the highlight of my entire career. Gene Wilburn wrote a story about the occasion. I will let him tell it:

> Dr. Frederick Chesley Elliott is a man of contrast. Although a dentist he heads the state's largest medical facility, the $110 million Texas Medical Center. He is also an accomplished cook. Despite culinary ability with steaks, chops, salads, and a charcoal grill; however, Dr. Elliott is most proud of his coffee. Here, too, the man is unique. He roasts, grinds, and blends his own coffee. The key to these operations is described by friends as a contraption that looks like a revolving squirrel cage with a thermostat.
>
> A youthful 65, Dr. Elliott has been executive director of the Texas Medical Center since 1952. He was one of the founders. [His career] started with his graduation from the Kansas City Western Dental College (now the University of Missouri School of Dentistry). He

was a practicing dentist for a few years, with an office in the Kansas City Argyle Building, and also served as instructor at Kansas City Western Dental College.

Dr. Elliott married the former Ann Orr of Kansas City in 1928. He is a man to whom recognition is not strange. He had been honored by the medical and dental professions on several occasions, and has been recognized as a leader in Houston's health fields for nearly 30 years. He was lauded by the Houston District Dental Society at a special testimony in 1955. Dr. Elliott was named 'Man of the Year' by the alumni of the University of Kansas City College of Dentistry in 1954, headed a 14-member state committee to survey Texas facilities and programs for research and training in mental health, and has served on the state and city boards of health.

Dr. Elliott became a Houstonian in 1932, when he was named dean of the Texas Dental College—a forerunner of the University of Texas Dental Branch, now located in the Texas Medical Center. He previously had served as instructor at Kansas City-Western Dental College University of Kansas City School of Dentistry, and as head of Dental Prosthesis department at the University of Tennessee.

The University of Texas took over the Texas Dental College in 1943 and Dr. Elliott was named its dean. Three years later he was elevated to a vice presidency of the University of Texas while retaining the deanship. That was the year the Texas Medical Center was actually started on a 134-acre tract adjoining Hermann Park. Prior to his appointment as executive-director of the Texas Medical Center, Dr. Elliott had served as its secretary and a member of the board.

Earlier this year he was named executive secretary of the newly formed Joint Administrative Committee of the Texas Medical Center and the Baylor University College of Medicine. He has been termed by associates, 'A man who can dream—then make the dreams come true.' Dr. Elliott was born in Pittsburgh, Kansas in 1893. He and his wife, Ann, live at 2345 Quenby.

Whew! This is a verbatim copy of Gene's story that appeared in the *Houston Chronicle* on May 17. As usual, some small errors are contained, and as I read it, I wondered how Gene got so much information. While one should appreciate the recognition of his accomplishments, it is always a little embarrassing to read an account of them in a prominent newspaper.[11]

Through the years, recognition came not only to the Medical Center, but also to many of the outstanding scientists who had come from other institutions to become a part of our center. This was the case with an outstanding faculty member from Tulane University School of Medicine who came to our Medical Center as the Judson Taylor Professor of Surgery—Dr. Michael DeBakey. On June 10, 1959, Dr. DeBakey received one of the most treasured medical awards given in the United States—the American Medical Association's Distinguished Service Medal. Dr. DeBakey was the first Texan to receive the award and the fourth to receive it in the entire South. Recognition such as this, bestowed upon our Medical Center scientists, brought high honor to all of us.

Saturday, July 11, 1959, was a heartwarming day for those of us who had dreamed of someday seeing an institution in our Medical Center that was devoted to the study and research of mental illness. Ground was finally broken for the new Houston State Institute for Research and Training. Dr. C. Ruilman, newly appointed head of the state hospital system, and Dr. William Lhamon, proudly presented their plans for the operation of the institute at the ceremonies. Dr. Lhamon was the new professor of psychiatry at Baylor University College of Medicine. I was the principal speaker for the occasion.

Another expansion program happened at the Medical Center. Dr. Lee Clark, on October 7, 1959, announced the plan to add seventy thousand more square feet of building space for research. He anticipated that it would cost between $2.5 million and $3 million. This expansion was to double the original space allocated for research in the M. D. Anderson Hospital and Tumor Institute. I believe that the accumulation of knowledge is infinite, and there are always unknowns that need to be discovered. More facilities would always be required to house the scientists and their instruments who maybe one day would find the answer to the difficult question, "What is cancer?" And on October 12, Dr. Lee Clark became president of the alumni association of the Mayo Foundation, a rather a small and select group. Those selected by the foundation as fellows were highly recommended by their alma mater. This was, again, another great honor for our center.

Should I mention the city-county hospital difficulties again? This time it was a money problem that developed between the city and county officials. On October 12, a newspaper headline read: "Early Start on Hospital Faces Fresh Obstacles." The county officials, possibly fearful of losing political prestige, did not want to release the six million dollars that they were holding for construction of the hospital. They said that their objections to releasing the funds were based on the assumption that the federal government would have "too much say," as one commissioner put it, in the operation of the hospital. Another commissioner commented, "The city councilmen and the mayor would get all the credit." This fear should have been allayed by a later statement from Mayor Cutrer when he said, "It is immaterial to me whether they put their money with ours or we put our money with theirs. We can handle it anyway the county wants it handled." Still, there were no announcements that the hospital would begin construction in the Medical Center any time soon.[12]

On October 16, the Rockefeller Foundation awarded a grant of ten thousand dollars to the Institute of Religion. To this sum, the Anderson Foundation added an additional five thousand dollars. These two grants were to support a four-year clinical study of the mental attitudes of heart and cancer patients. The institute was making endeavors in the study of spiritual relations to mental attitudes in times of stress.

As related earlier, the Medical Center was to be responsible for the funds to be used in the construction of a new building for Baylor University College of Medicine. On the first of November, Irvin Shenkler presented me with a check for $100,000 which was to apply to the $450,000 that had been pledged by the Jewish community to build a Jewish Medical Research Institute at the medical school. Hundreds of individuals in the Jewish community made this pledge, a pleasing example of group action for the good of all.[13]

We were quickly reaching our goal for the funding of the three buildings that were to be constructed at Baylor Medical College. On November 6, we were informed that a grant of $2,395,139 had been approved by the National Institutes of Health. This sum was the full amount that we had requested for the medical college buildings. It was to match the $2.45 million grant that had been previously made to the Medical Center.

Quickly following the groundbreaking for the State Psychiatric Institute was the groundbreaking for the Institute of Religion. It was announced that the institute would be affiliated with all the theological seminaries in the state of Texas. This gave recognition to the Institute of Religion as an approved educational institution. Those who completed the course of study in the institute would receive credit from the seminaries toward the awarding of graduate degrees.[14]

On December 12, 1959, an article appeared in the *Houston Post* quoting an announcement by T. W. Weston, a Houston business consultant and representative for the Medical Center Monorail, that a monorail study was under way. The Medical Center Monorail was a limited partnership company. Weston, who had hopes that the monorail system in the Medical Center would be approved, mentioned that his company had spent some six months on the study of a monorail. As I mentioned earlier, his hopes for the monorail system in the Medical Center were to be dashed to the ground.

During the latter part of December, a grant of $125,000 was made to Baylor University College of Medicine by the Fondren Foundation for the support of research in ophthalmology in the new eye institute, which later occupied a portion of the Jewish Medical Research Institute building. At the time, the eye institute was operating in the Baldwin Street property—the former temporary quarters for the M. D. Anderson Hospital. The Texas Medical Center loaned this facility to Baylor University for the eye institute.[15]

A very busy 1959 came to a close on a sad note. Dr. Claude C. Cody, Jr., died on December 31. Dr. Cody played a very important part in making a medical library possible for the Medical Center. The medical community and the Medical Center had lost another friend and great leader.[16]

Expansion, Innovation, and Retirement, 1960–63

POLIO WAS ONE OF THE MOST dreaded diseases that plagued human beings until the successful introduction of the Salk vaccine in 1955. The Salk vaccine was hailed as a godsend at the time it was introduced, and it was. The death rate and the crippling of victims by polio dropped dramatically after its introduction. Though the use of the Salk vaccine had decreased the number of poliomyelitis cases between eighty-five and ninety percent, there was still a margin of anxiety of ten percent. Dr. Albert Sabin, professor of research pediatrics at the University of Cincinnati, developed a new type of vaccine, a "live virus" that could be given by mouth.[1]

It was early in January, 1960, that Dr. Joseph Melnick, professor of virology at Baylor University College of Medicine, began a series of studies with this new vaccine. Two hundred and fifty children were to be given a one dose vaccination by mouth. The purpose was to determine to what extent the "wild" vaccine might serve to immunize other family members that the child came in contact with. The wild vaccine was a type of immunity that caused the development of a similar type of immunity when it was passed from one individual to another. Some thirteen million children in several different nations, including Russia, had received the vaccine. This was the first in our city and additional field studies were to be conducted in other cities as well. If these field studies proved to be effective it was expected that the Salk vaccine would be released for general use. As we later found out, it was the beginning of the end of the ravages caused by the polio virus. A $170,855 grant had been made by a national foundation to Dr. Melnick for this study. It was another expression of recognition for our Medical Center.[2]

On January 11, another grant was announced for Baylor College of Medicine. Texaco awarded a grant of one hundred thousand dollars to the medical school for the support of research and education. Though not generally known, companies like Texaco were making sizable grants to educational and research institutions each year. Then the National Institutes of Health announced that five grants had been made to scientists in our Medical Center for different purposes. The rapid increase in the number of grants meant a great deal to the founders of the Medical Center and assured them that their vision had been sound. While the gifts from the large foundations were huge at the time they were given, the trustees were more rewarded by the returns they received from the thousands of patients who had been treated. How many lives that have been saved, no one knows. From a financial point of view, each year the funds that were expended for the operation of the institutions in the Medical Center exceeded the total amount of the grants that were received for buildings.

It is unfortunate that the city-county hospital affair was such a bitter, personal controversy. It stifled the usual progressive programs of the medical professional meetings. On January 14, 1960, when the Harris County Medical Society installed new officers, Dr. Robert W. Kimbro, president of the Texas Medical Association, took the society to task at the banquet given for the new officers. While he did not aim his remarks to all the members of the society present, he did say that "sometimes there are strong-minded individuals who feel that they should dominate the medical scene in the community and they're only willing to cooperate when it suits their whim and fancy." Dr. Kimbro continued by saying, "I personally do not feel that there is any place for an individual or a group of individuals in a medical society, medical school, or a teaching institution who are willing to undermine the prestige and standing of his professional colleagues in a community simply by being selfish or hard-headed." There must have been several red faces on some who listened to these timely and worthwhile criticisms. Some of the prominent leaders in the medical society had previously made the same criticisms in person to the individuals that Dr. Kimbro was fingering. At the same meeting, Dr. Wendell Hamrick was elected president of the Harris County Medical Society. In his remarks following the announcement of his election, Dr. Hamrick voiced sentiments in line with Dr. Kimbro's "scolding." When asked by a reporter later, Dr. Hamrick commented on Kimbro's address, stating, "He wasn't passing out any compliments." The personal animosity did not abate.

On February 19, the Anderson Foundation announced that a grant of $500,000 had been made to St. Joseph's Hospital to help in their endeavor to enlarge their facilities for patient care. We were pleased with the announcement. From the beginning of the Medical Center it had been hoped that more and better citywide health care facilities would develop so that the Medical Center could be of better service to the people of Houston and Harris County. This was the wish of Monroe D. Anderson and the trustees of the Anderson Foundation were seeing to it that his wishes were being fulfilled. St. Joseph's Hospital, like the Veteran's Hospital and Baptist Hospital (later Memorial), all were serving as Medical Center satellite hospitals for teaching and research for the medical school, the dental school, and the postgraduate school of medicine.[3]

More and more the Medical Center was demonstrating its growth to maturity by increasing research and educational activities. On February 21, the University of Texas Postgraduate School of Medicine gave a postgraduate symposium. Nineteen guest speakers brought new medical information for the physicians who attended the three-day conference. Physicians came from many of the nearby counties and smaller communities. I was pleased to learn that Dr. Viktor E. Frankl, professor of neurology and psychiatry of the University of Vienna, had accepted the invitation of Dr. William Lhamon, chairman of the department of psychiatry at Baylor University College of Medicine, to lecture in Houston. I had visited the University of Vienna in 1936 when Dr. Frankl was a young man in the medical school. Dr. Gottlieb, professor of pathology of the university, introduced me to him.[4]

Dr. Frankl was to become an outstanding man in his field. His lectures in Houston did not follow the same philosophy of life expressed by one he knew in Vienna, Dr. Sigmund Freud. Dr. Frankl lectured to three different groups: the faculty of the psychiatric department of Baylor College of Medicine and students at the school, the Texas Medical Center Research Society, and one lecture was given to the public. Dr. Frankl's name was a familiar one in the circles of psychologists and psychiatrists, and his books were widely read. Dr. Frankl's words from his lectures would serve well even today. In one of his remarks he said, "Alcoholism, juvenile delinquency, anxieties, obsessions, and so forth, were due some to the individual not sensing an awareness of life's worthwhileness." This, he thought, should be replaced by getting the individual to understand and know his own purpose in life, then devoting his energies to achieving that goal.

Since it was the first of its kind in the Medical Center, the Institute of Religion was to be confronted with the difficulties of a pioneer. First, there was puzzlement about its purpose in the Medical Center and how it might be possible to do research in the field. Second, and most important, was funding for its building and its support. Building funds, though not as readily accumulated as they were for illnesses like heart disease and cancer, were given to the board for the construction of the building. Through the years, though, difficulties would arise when funds were sought for operating expenses, research, and teaching. The institute was not an organized church. It had no congregation on which it could depend for support, so its funds had to come from gifts and grants. On February 26, 1960, Houston Endowment, Inc., the foundation established by Jesse H. Jones, made a grant of one hundred thousand dollars to the Institute of Religion for its building, which was under construction at the time. Dr. Dawson Bryan, director of the institute, when expressing his appreciation for the grant, pointed out that the Institute of Religion had been operating in the Medical Center in temporary quarters in the Jesse H. Jones Library building since 1955. Classes were conducted as workshop programs in the hospitals and in the medical school. In explaining the purpose of the institute, he also mentioned how the plan began. "A group of men here in the Texas Medical Center are treating patients with a new kind of medicine," he said. "They are ministering to the soul. They are chaplain interns from the Institute of Religion, learning to provide the sick with pastoral care. Man's enemy is not alone the microbe, but also himself," Dr. Bryan explained. "Thus, the concept of healing the whole person—spiritually, as well as mentally and physically, is accomplished." He continued by saying, "It was Dr. Fred Elliott's idea, but he won't take credit for it."[5]

While the first contacts for such a program emanated from my office, the concept of research and teaching in the area of religion began at Methodist Hospital. Clyde Verheyden, director of religious activities in the hospital, had conducted several seminars for ministers who served hospitals as part-time chaplains and for pastors who visited members of their congregations who were hospital patients. Verheyden had brought several outstanding lecturers in pastoral care to Houston to conduct the seminars. Dr. Bryan had been a resident of Houston for twenty-one years. He served as pastor of St. Paul's Methodist Church for ten years before becoming a co-pastor at First Methodist Church. I became acquainted with Dr. Bryan when I arrived in Houston. It was in his church, St. Paul's, where we held our graduation exercises. Dr. Bryan always gave the baccalaureate sermons. He did not have the opportunity to serve the institute for too long a time.

During March, we were saddened to learn that one of our prominent professors, Dr. Fred Bloom, had died. He had served as a clinical professor at the Baylor University College of Medicine. Dr. Bloom's death was sudden; he died on the golf course. He had reached the fifteenth tee when his heart decided it had had enough. It was a fatal heart attack. A death such as this, at the age of fifty-six, always causes me to be somewhat critical of physicians for neglecting their own health.

In the early part of April, we learned that the first associate dean of Texas Woman's University School of Nursing in our Medical Center had been selected. Kathryn Crossland was to arrive in late June. She would be very busy, since her first class was to begin in September. In the meantime, a faculty had to be selected, the curriculum planned, and clinical teaching programs organized. Crossland, at the time, was director of nursing at the University of Alabama.

It is only natural that I was pleased when I heard of honors going to the scientists in our Medical Center for their outstanding contributions in the field of research. On April 27, we learned that the College of France had chosen Dr. Roger Guillemin to be the recipient for the Prix Saintour. Only three years earlier Dr. Guillemin had received the Louis Boneau Award. He was now to divide his time between the faculty of the College of France in Paris and Baylor University College of Medicine.[6]

Recognition of the quality of professional education and research at our Medical Center came fast compared to the usual amount of time it took for many other major educational centers in the United States. Another example of this rapid progress was Dr. Murray Copeland's acceptance of an appointment as assistant director for education at the University of Texas M. D. Anderson Hospital and Tumor Institute. Dr. Copeland was chairman of the department of oncology at Georgetown University Medical Center in Washington, D.C. He was internationally known in the field of oncology and had been awarded an honorary doctor of science degree from Oglethorpe University. Indeed, the Texas Medical Center continued to be extremely fortunate in the way that top-level medical scientists accepted staff and faculty appointments at our institutions.

Finally, on May 22, 1960, we celebrated another groundbreaking. Mr. and Mrs. Newton Rayzor had made a grant of $300,000 for the construction of a student center. The Rayzor Student Center was to be the connecting link between the Jones and Anderson buildings and later would be adjoined by the Jewish Research Institute. Dr. Michael DeBakey, in the few remarks that he made, stated that many lives might be saved in the future by the fruit of the research endeavors to be conducted in these Baylor research facilities.[7]

On May 22, 1960, the fifteenth anniversary year of the Medical Center, the Anderson Foundation released a report. It was an outstanding example of what could be done with private endowment funds when they were expertly managed and not hampered or "hamstrung" by federal regulations. In 1942, the M. D. Anderson Foundation received almost all of the estate of Monroe D. Anderson, who had died on August 6, 1939. The Anderson Foundation received about nineteen million dollars.

Since then, the Anderson Foundation authorized grants amounting to $23,069,103 by the time the report was written in 1960. Had the capital funds of the foundation been granted during this time, the foundation would have been in the red a sizable amount. The foundation, in 1960, had a book value of $28,550,000. The grants that the foundation made since its founding were detailed in the report. It is a must that such accomplishments not be forgotten, and for people not to conclude that this is the present-day accumulated accomplishment of the foundation. Grants have been made since this date in 1960, and, in spite of government regulations, the trustees of the foundation have continued to increase the book value of the foundation's assets.

The foundation made grants to several other universities, including Rice Institute, the University of Houston, the University of Texas, Texas A&M College, St. Thomas University, and the Harding College in Searcy, Arkansas. In addition to these grants to colleges and universities, there were also grants given to programs for other activities in the city of Houston such as to the YMCA for their new Negro Branch, their downtown branch, and the north side branch; to the Boy Scouts; and to the Salvation Army. Several smaller amounts that the foundation gave were not listed in the report. However, the first grant made by the Anderson Foundation was made to the Junior League for the purchase of eyeglasses for poor children.[8]

To see a compilation of grants made to the Medical Center and its institutions by other foundations in Houston would be most worthwhile. Another grant I want to mention again is the one made by Marshall G. Johnson and his wife to the Lutheran Hospital Association for the construction of the Lutheran Hospital in the Texas Medical Center. The University of Texas M. D. Anderson Hospital and Tumor Institute would operate the hospital. The seventeen million dollar grant was the largest grant ever to be received by the University of Texas or any institution in the Medical Center at the time I write this. As John Freeman, chairman of the Anderson Foundation at the time the report was released, remarked, "We have a definite plan in spending this money. We try to get something rolling and encourage others to help." Ample proof of the wisdom in this statement abounds throughout Houston.

With as many times that I have mentioned groundbreaking exercises in the Medical Center, one might think that there would not be another square foot of ground to be broken. Yet there was. 1960 was a boom year for groundbreaking. Methodist Hospital groundbreaking exercises were held on Wednesday, June 1, 1960, for their new nine million dollar expansion program. Mrs. Walter W. Fondren, one of the largest donors, turned the first spade of dirt, even though she was confined to a wheelchair following a recent illness. Three hundred and seventy-five beds were to be added to the hospital. When the addition was completed, seven hundred beds would be available for patient care as well as expanded facilities for surgery. O'Bannion Williams, chairman of the board of trustees of the Methodist Hospital, presided at the ceremonies.[9]

On June 3, 1960, the largest single grant to be received in the Medical Center up to this time, 124,000 shares of Anderson, Clayton & Company stock, was given by Mrs. W. L. Clayton to establish an endowment fund for Texas Children's Hospital. The stock was valued at the time at over $4.5 million. A reporter questioned me concerning this grant, and I informed him that, "The value of such philanthropy as this is too great to determine its worth. It means an expanded program by the hospital, especially in research. There isn't any ceiling on research."[10]

Another groundbreaking on June 7 was for the new Jewish Research Institute. This was one of the four buildings built for Baylor University College of Medicine by funds given to the Medical Center and also by a large federal grant. Dr. Bernard Farfel was the principal speaker. In his remarks Dr. Farfel said, "All through the Torah, the Jewish Bible, there are references to healing. It is the Jewish encyclopedia of medicine." Dr. Farfel then said, "It is the belief that the person who saves one life saves the world." It was this belief that prompted the Jewish community to raise $450,000 toward the construction of the building. The research completed in this building through the years has more than justified Dr. Farfel's remarks.[11]

On June 30, it was announced that Isaac Arnold, a son-in-law of Roy Cullen, was to head a drive for a nine million dollar expansion program for St. Luke's Hospital. Expansion plans for buildings in the Medical Center were continually being announced. The funds expended for the buildings completed far exceeded the amounts needed at the time the expansion plans were announced.

In August, two long serving Medical Center stalwarts—Dr. Roy C. Heflebower, assistant director of M. D. Anderson Hospital and Tumor Institute, and Miss Anna Hanselman, who had been with the cancer hospital from the beginning—announced that they were retiring on September 1. To those of us who had worked with Miss Hanselman when the hospital was but a dream, it seemed that she was a permanent part of our Medical Center structure. For Miss Hanselman and for us it was a regrettable realization that time waits for no one. Later in September, at a meeting of the board of regents of the University of Texas, an addition to M. D. Anderson Hospital and Tumor Institute was approved that would provide more research space. It was estimated that the addition would cost $4.3 million.[12]

On October 2, Dr. Stanley Olson announced that the first heart research center would be established at Baylor University College of Medicine. The institute plan had been developed by the medical school and approved by the National Heart Institute of the United States Public Health Service. The first year's appropriation was $262,500, the second year the appropriation would be increased to $396,350, then to $491,325 for each of the years thereafter through to the eighth year.[13]

On October 30, the American Cancer Society announced that a lifetime research grant would be made to Dr. A. Clark Griffin, head of the biochemistry department at the University of Texas M. D. Anderson Hospital and Tumor Institute. Dr. Griffin's project was long-range, therefore, this grant made it possible for him to feel secure in the knowledge that his research would be supported throughout his life.[14]

The year 1960 was a most satisfactory one. Construction started on building after building while research grants were increasing rapidly in number. Thirty-seven sizable grants for research were received by the various institutions in the Medical Center, each for some project that engaged a number of individuals. Discoveries were yet to be made, some that would be life saving and others that would be disappointing. But this huge enterprise, the Texas Medical Center, as its name implies, was a center for all of Texas and the world where research was the chief enterprise.

The year 1961 may be regarded as a year of review since some plans that had been proposed earlier were now being restudied. Also it was a year in which several innovations would be announced. In February, a booklet called "Television Facilities," published by the University of Texas Dental Branch, described in detail how television was being used for teaching in the dental school. Widespread interest in the University of Texas Dental Branch television facilities had generated many requests for information regarding the program. Earl Morrison, director of the television facilities, had developed methods for the use of television in teaching. In the book he described the studies that were done and the equipment that was used. The difficulties that Morrison encountered when using television as a teaching media in the dental school prompted him to develop many new types of equipment. Close-up views of a single tooth in the mouth were among the problems that he had to solve. The television equipment available was not suitable. Also, dental surgeons had to develop new methods for operating so that arms and fingers would not block the view of the camera lens while he was operating. Morrison developed two new types of cameras. One was the ultra close-up camera, and the second one was an intra-oral or "in the mouth" camera. Extraordinary pictures were possible with these cameras. The booklet described the equipment that was developed in detail so that other teaching institutions could use it. Cameras could be used for teaching in other fields of education, too. Later, Morrison developed a television microscope. It was a miraculous and complicated piece of equipment. He also began developing a difficult type of teaching equipment—the three dimensional camera.

On February 4, 1961, the board for Texas State Hospitals and Special Schools announced the opening of the Houston State Psychiatric Hospital in the Medical Center. The chairman of the board stated in his address, "Now Texas has one of the world's most modern psychiatric institutes, with a staff of respected scientists, teachers and clinicians, representing many professions gathered together in the interest of a common goal." It was a day that had been made possible because of Governor Allan Shivers's keen interest in the serious problem of mental disease that confronted the state. It was his action that had prompted the 55th legislature of the state to establish the state psychiatric institute. Dr. T. Lhamon was the first director.

At the annual dinner of the Pierre Fauchard Academy held in Chicago on February 4, 1961, I received the twenty-fourth Fauchard Gold Medal. In presenting the award, Dr. Thomas P. Fox of Philadelphia, president of the academy, read the citation: "Awarded for distinguished contributions to dentistry and health sciences as an educator, planner, and administrator."

At a meeting of the board of trustees of the Texas Medical Center on March 7, Colonel Bates made a motion, which was approved, to refer the Fred Buxton and Associates report to the executive committee for action. The "Buxton Report" was based upon a study that Buxton had made concerning the growing traffic problem in the Medical Center. A lady named Mrs. McAshan was interested in beautifying the grounds of the Medical Center—she was concerned about the appearance of the parking lots and wanted more restful areas of trees and flowers to take their place. She elicited the interest of her father, Will Clayton, in the project. It was her recommendation that prompted the board of the Medical Center to engage Buxton in the study. Buxton's proposal was interesting since he suggested lowering all streets in the Medical Center to a depth that would allow pedestrian traffic to cross over on walkways slightly above ground level. Likewise, the seven garages that he proposed would be at the lowered street level with another level above. The upper level over the second level of parking would have been sodded and trees planted to provide the beauty spots Mrs. Mc-Ashan so desired. Booths (kiosks) were to be built at each entrance and a fee would be collected for parking in the Medical Center. Buxton's proposal was not accepted. However, when paid parking in the Medical Center became a reality, the kiosks were built.

At the same meeting of the board of trustees, a request was made by Methodist Hospital for the construction of a tunnel under Wilkins Avenue, which had been proposed much earlier. The tunnel would have connected Methodist Hospital with properties north of it. However, engineering studies revealed that it was not possible to construct a tunnel because of the underground utilities that lay under Wilkins Avenue. Also, some of the main storm sewers draining the Medical Center had been placed under the street.

At the close of 1961, on December 13, I received a letter from the Ellerbe Company in Minneapolis, Minnesota, suggesting that I join their company in a consulting capacity. I was somewhat surprised since I had not made my intentions publicly known that I was planning on retiring my appointment as director of the Texas Medical Center. It was a rewarding offer since I felt that the request demonstrated a degree of confidence in my ability for planning. Later, I learned that the Southwest Medical Foundation in San Antonio had informed Ellerbe that I had been serving them in this capacity. I declined the invitation to join the Ellerbe staff.

A rather tranquil 1961 was drawing to a close. An agreement finally had been reached between the city of Houston and Harris County to build the city-county hospital in the Medical Center. At the hospital groundbreaking exercises it was announced that the hospital would be called the Ben Taub Hospital, in honor of the man who had served so many years as the chairman of the Harris County Charity Hospital board of managers.

Early in 1962, it was time that I should make plans to retire. I had begun discussing my desire to relinquish my appointment as full-time director of the Texas Medical Center much earlier. First, I discussed my plan with Leland Anderson, and then with other members of the board of trustees. When I first mentioned my desire to Anderson he seemed quite reluctant to accept my decision. He asked me to reconsider and give it some more thought before I made a final move. I told him that it was my feeling that the Medical Center was entering into a period that would require the energies of one much younger than I. At a later meeting with Anderson, I suggested a plan to him that I had given considerable thought. I felt that the Medical Center needed to have more input with its institutions so that it would be much easier to coordinate the relationships between them. I be-

lieved that it was a good time to get the plan underway. I suggested to Anderson that the Medical Center establish a development office similar to the
one of the University of Texas. I told Anderson that we should continue to
search for a full-time director, but that I could continue on a half-time basis
as director of the Medical Center development program. At the time a new
director was appointed, I explained to Anderson that the director for development would serve with the board in developing plans that would be submitted to the board of trustees for their approval. Also, I explained that the
development office should be located somewhere in the downtown section
near his office, since the director for development would be under the supervision of the Medical Center's board. This plan was presented to the
board of trustees and approved. A development committee of the Medical
Center's board was appointed.

I suggested to the board that since several of the institutions had changed
the title of their administrators to that of vice president, that the new director of the Texas Medical Center should be named an executive vice president. The board authorized me to search for the right person. I contacted
several individuals for the appointment, one of whom was Dr. Richard T.
Eastwood, vice president of the University of Alabama. At the time, he was
the officer in charge of business operations for the University of Alabama in
Birmingham. The medical center campus of the University of Alabama was
located in Birmingham. When Dr. Eastwood came to Houston to discuss
the appointment with me, I was impressed with his friendly manner and his
grasp of medical center affairs. His education in business administration and
his background and experience with the University of Alabama seemed to
fit him well for the vice presidency of the Texas Medical Center. Dr. Eastwood also visited with Leland Anderson and some of the administrators at
that time.

The first meeting of the board of trustees for the year was held on January 26, 1962. Several items of routine business were considered, among
which were several change orders for the buildings that were being constructed by the Medical Center for Baylor University College of Medicine.
I reported to the board that the parking plan was still under discussion. Several meetings had been held with the council of administrators.

Some faculty members of Baylor's Department of Preventive Medicine,
had discussed with me the possibility of locating the Houston public health
department in the Medical Center. A building for the city health department had been under consideration for some time. The members of the executive committee of the Medical Center were familiar with the idea since it

had been informally discussed previously. At the meeting of the board, I took time to impress them with the importance of having the building in the Medical Center. First, it would serve to arouse more interest in the approval of the public health school of the University of Texas, which was planned for the Medical Center. I explained that it would serve the public health school in the same manner that a hospital serves the medical school. My reason for asking for board action at this time was based upon a move that was underway to locate the building for the public health department in the civic center downtown. The public health officer and the faculty of the department of Preventative Medicine at the medical school felt that this would be a serious mistake. It would have prevented the health department from securing grants for research from the United States Public Health Service. Also, the faculties of the Dental Branch and the medical school and the public health school would waste considerable time traveling back and forth between the civic center and the Medical Center. While the board took no formal action, several members of the board stated that they would make the proper contacts with city officials.

The meeting of the executive committee held on March 6, 1962, was devoted entirely to a lengthy discussion of the plan for a controlled parking program for the Medical Center. I had been interviewing candidates for the manager of the Medical Center parking. The parking garage, which was to be purchased by the Medical Center from Methodist Hospital, and the operation of the parking lots in the Center, would require a full-time person. All parking lots in the whole complex would be supervised by the Medical Center. The parking lots at the time were being operated by each individual institution. I explained to the executive committee members that it was essential that all institutions in the Medical Center agree to the plan, otherwise it would not be possible to convert all entrances to the Medical Center into paid entrances, but Methodist Hospital and Hermann Hospital administrators raised some objections. Finally the executive committee decided that the parking and traffic committee of the board of trustees of the Medical Center should meet with the council of administrators. Dr. Eastwood's appointment also was discussed briefly at this meeting. Leland Anderson was asked to write to Dr. Eastwood, requesting that he make another trip to Houston for further discussions concerning the appointment.

At the executive committee meeting of the Medical Center held on April 4, several routine business matters were considered. Colonel Bates, the newly appointed chairman of the development committee that had been appointed earlier, reported on a meeting with Dr. Grant Taylor. Dr. Taylor was chairman of a special committee of the University of Texas institutions in the Medical Center. He reported to Colonel Bates and the development committee that the university was planning a building on the tract of ground west of the dental school building, a parking lot at the time. The building was to be a large facility of several floors. It would contain an underground garage that would house two thousand vehicles. The aboveground tower structure would provide quarters for the Postgraduate School of Medicine, the School of Industrial and Environmental Medicine, a communication center, a large auditorium with a seating capacity of twenty-five hundred, and resident facilities for continuation and graduate students. This was another attempt for such a facility that failed.

Following Colonel Bates's report, a somewhat lengthy conversation developed concerning a request by Methodist Hospital for an additional four acres of land. At the time the request was made, Methodist Hospital did not indicate any use for the land. Since land was in short supply, I suggested to the trustees that land should not be allocated or deeded to any institution existing or contemplated until a definite need for the land was demonstrated and that the preliminary architectural plans be submitted to the architectural committee for their approval. Action on the request was delayed and the board of trustees of Methodist Hospital was informed of this action.

Anderson was then asked to express the appreciation of the trustees to Newton Gresham for the part that he had played in obtaining an insurance company settlement of $13,023 for the damage that Hurricane Carla had caused to a Texas Woman's University building. The storm had also caused considerable damage to the trees in the Medical Center, creating a rather devastated appearance. Over 150 trees had been downed by the storm. At the time we had only two grounds employees, and they were slowly clearing the downed trees and cutting them into fireplace lengths. Our part-time grounds supervisor and I felt that these could be sold. But we learned that because of Hurricane Carla, fireplace wood was in abundance. We gave the firewood to anyone who would remove it. I informed the trustees of this action and added that Will Clayton and Mrs. McAshan were still interested in a beautification plan for the Medical Center. I was asked to express the appreciation of the trustees for their continued interest but to inform Mrs. McAshan that the beautification program would be delayed until the buildings under construction in the Medical Center had been completed.

Just prior to adjournment of the meeting, Leland Anderson announced that Dr. Eastwood had informed him that he would accept the appointment as executive vice president of the Texas Medical Center. He was to begin his appointment on August 15, 1962. Since my term as full-time executive director of the Medical Center was quickly drawing to a close, I had requested several executive committee meetings so that action could be taken on pending projects that I had recommended. On May 4 and 7, meetings were held. The meeting on May 4 was for the purpose of receiving the report of the parking and grounds committee. The committee chairman reported that since the majority of the institutions had approved the parking plan, that plans should be made to close the entrances to the Medical Center after the construction of the kiosks had been completed. Hermann Hospital was the only hospital that was reluctant to enter into this plan since the major portion of their parking lot faced Outer Belt Drive. Favrot reported that the Medical Center must either lease or purchase the Methodist Hospital garage. It was decided later to purchase it. The Anderson Foundation provided the funds for the purchase.

In May, the new officers for the Medical Center were selected. Leland Anderson was re-elected as president; Col. William B. Bates, Hines Baker, and I were elected vice presidents; Dr. Richard T. Eastwood was elected executive vice president and secretary of the board of trustees; and William Kirkland and Carroll Simmons were re-elected to the offices of treasurer and assistant treasurer. Dr. Eastwood was present at the meeting and expressed his pleasure in being identified with the Medical Center.

In the early part of June, Dr. Victor Olson, dean of the University of Texas Dental Branch, invited me to be the commencement speaker for their graduation. I recall that I spoke on the subject of values. As commencement addresses go, as far as the graduates are concerned, it was the usual, run-of-the-mill address. I reminded the graduates of this in my opening remarks when I said, "If one were to lay commencement day speakers end to end, this would be just about right." I think I saw a few nods of approval at this remark. It was a nice day for Ann and me. It had been just ten years since I had been present at the last graduation of the Dental Branch, at the time I was dean of the dental school. Dr. Olson had planned a surprise for us. He gave a luncheon for Ann and me immediately following the graduation exercises. After the luncheon, with faculty and friends present, he had a portrait of me unveiled. This was the first time that Ann and I saw the portrait. We deeply appreciated the thoughtfulness of Dr. Olson in having this portrait done. As wives usually do Ann commented, "It doesn't do you justice."

On July 31, 1962, I was to present my final agenda to the Medical Center's board of trustees. Since so many actions had been taken at the executive meetings that required the approval of the board of trustees, it was a lengthy meeting. John Jones reported on the progress that was being made for the construction of the building for Texas Woman's University College of Nursing. The contract had been awarded. Also, Jones reported that since another building was under consideration, which would house male students from Baylor University College of Medicine, the University of Texas Dental Branch, as well as graduate students, that the plans for the power plant had been delayed. The committee felt that one power plant could be provided that would serve both buildings. This would eliminate the need for dual facilities, as well as reduce to a considerable degree the cost of operation. Jones informed the trustees that sufficient funds were available for the purchase of furnishings for March Culmore Hall. Also, Jones reported on a conversation with Dr. Guinn, president of Texas Woman's University. Dr. Guinn believed that it was essential that the College of Nursing in the Medical Center begin a graduate nursing educational program as early as possible. Dr. Guinn wanted the Texas Medical Center's board of trustees to approve such a program so that it would lend emphasis to the request that the university planned to make in October to the Commission on Higher Education for approval of the program.

The trustees were also advised of the last executive committee meeting, when concerns about the availability of land for future building were voiced. Following this discussion, Leland Anderson was requested to discuss with the parking and grounds committee the content of a letter that should be mailed to the trustees of each institution in the Medical Center. The letter would inform them that land would no longer be allocated until plans for the programs were discussed and approved, and also that the architectural elevations be submitted to the board of trustees for referral to the architectural committee. Finally, the board of trustees approved an instrument that would allow Hermann Hospital to continue using the land that was the property of the Medical Center which they had been using since their new addition had been constructed. Following this action, the board adjourned. My next presence at a Texas Medical Center Board of Trustees meeting was as an officer of the board, and not as the director.

When I informed my only two office employees that I was retiring, they told me that they would seek employment elsewhere. Their reasons were valid. They believed that Dr. Eastwood would wish to employ those that worked closely with him. Mollie Halmark, my secretary, obtained employment elsewhere in the early part of the year and left the Medical Center office, effective June 1, 1962. Rosalie Levinson, my stenographer, remained with me until August 14, the day before Dr. Eastwood's arrival. I moved my office into my former secretary's office. Miss Levinson and I had prepared my former office for Dr. Eastwood's arrival.

A new period in my life was to begin as director for development. This was a half-time appointment. After Dr. Eastwood's arrival, we spent some time together discussing the various projects that were underway. Dr. Eastwood needed very little information from me since he had devoted the first few weeks to reviewing the various projects under construction and to studying the material in the office. He also visited with the administrators of the institutions in the Medical Center and discussed with them their programs as they related to the center. I began giving some thought to the plans for developing a funding program. I had developed what I thought would be a satisfactory plan. I asked the stenographer to type the plan and have it ready for me when I returned from a short vacation that Ann and I had planned.

Late in 1960, Ann and I had purchased an Airstream travel trailer. We had made a few short trips to become acquainted with it and with this mode of travel. We left Houston in the fall of 1962 and made a trip in the trailer to the [Rio Grande] Valley for a short vacation. When I returned to the office after our vacation, I called Leland Anderson and informed him that I had returned. He asked that I come to his office when it was convenient for me to do so. I told him that it would be convenient the next morning. The next day, he informed me that during my absence, Dr. Eastwood had raised the question as to whether the development office should be a function of the board of trustees or whether it wouldn't be better to have it as a function of the administrative office. The executive committee considered this question, and it was decided that the development program should be an administrative function. Anderson informed me that I would now be working directly with Dr. Eastwood. I learned later that a similar action had been taken by the board of regents of the University of Texas and the university development Office was now a function of the president's office.

I presumed that this must have been one of the reasons why Hulon Black resigned as director of the development office of the University of Texas. I studied many different plans that I thought might be workable under the new arrangement. None of them were shown to Dr. Eastwood since I was not pleased with any of them. After some time, I decided that it would be best if I were to resign. This would permit Dr. Eastwood to make a plan for development that would be more satisfactory to him. I left the Medical Center as an employee on May 31, 1963. My many years of active work—fifty-three years in all—were over.

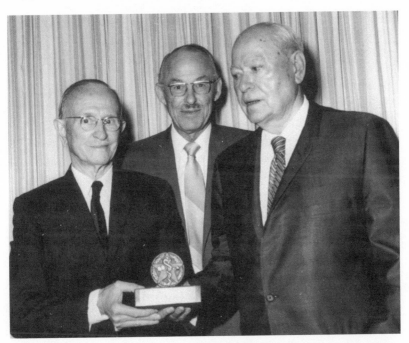

Elliott, Dr. R. Lee Clark, and Col. William B. Bates in 1970. The Texas Medical Center honored Elliott and Bates with a Medallion in recognition of their contributions as founders.

On June 4, Ann and I were on our way for a four-month trip through the eastern half of Canada. Several more lengthy trips throughout the United States were to follow. Upon our return from the trip to Canada, I found a letter awaiting me from the University of Kansas City (now University of Missouri of Kansas City), asking me to represent the president of the University of Kansas City at the inauguration of Dr. Kenneth S. Pitzer, the third president of William Marsh Rice University. This was a colorful event with presidents and representatives from universities throughout the United States, Canada, and Europe present. Each of us was given a bronze medal for being a participant in the inauguration. I also remained a member of the board of trustees of the Texas Medical Center, and through the years I have missed very few of the meetings.

As I lay my pen down I look across the desk at a letter that lies open. Reading it again a moment ago for the "nth" time, the notion came to my mind that the depth of feelings expressed in the letter are the only rewards that those who made the Medical Center possible need. It is fitting that I quote one or two paragraphs of this letter, which is from a mother who fought alongside the doctors a long, tiring battle to save the life of her young son— and lost.

> One day, in explaining the purpose of the Medical Center to me, you spoke of the whole man—physical, intellectual, and spiritual. You spoke of the aim to provide service, research, and education; the whole being equal to the sum of its parts. We realize that no part can be neglected if we are to reach the ultimate goal. Bricks and mortar touch the sky and pour forth miracles: mechanical heartbeats, toxins filter through clear tubes; the deaf hear; the blind see; and, the dying live—sometimes. The point is that man through study, application, and beneficence makes all of these things possible. Developing his talents, he is the tool, the inspiration, the foundation on which the monuments to his genius rest. Stand quietly, look around the Medical Center, and see the wonders that are before you. Gaze through the windows—what do you see that lives? You see the creation of God, man, and His world. Close your eyes. Block out the noise and concentrate. What do you feel? What do you sense stirring the air around you? Is it the striving of man? Is it a living force—an energy emanating as a collective wind of change from the efforts of the triangle that is man? It is. With all that is before us, it is man himself that is frequently overlooked. Man, the reason for our concern has sometimes been lost in the cause of disease and the eternal search for the solution. Like patriotism that falters when the rights of the individual are smothered. Specific pride for and support of the Medical Center falters when man, the individual is forced to identify with technology, rather than the ability of man himself makes it all work.
>
> The Medical Center means more to me today than it did before. It is true that the gift of a prolonged life for a beloved child left me grateful and with an appreciation of the quality of man, but it takes a lot of gratitude and admiration to cling to, in making myself 'keep on keeping on.' I sort of require constant transfusions of exposure to people that have those qualities of life that make what I call 'great men' for lack of a more descriptive word. It is more than accomplishments that I admire. It is the qualities that made them possible and the kind of person that shines through that cast their light for the rest of us. This is what the Medical Center is for me. It is those men who serve and treat the triangle of man—the whole man. It is men

of dedication and foresight; men whose ego spurs them on, men who dare to dream the impossible dream, men whose mistakes equal their triumphs, men of greatness who in their humility say, 'It was not I, but those who helped me.' They are men with a broad view that work for mankind, but leave for a legacy, bouquets of kindness and compassion, as well.

It is a difficult thing that I am trying to say. To have a clearer picture of what is our Medical Center, we need to know the men who are the Medical Center. We need to know the man behind the accomplishments, the man behind the discoveries and the announcements, the man that laughs and cries, the man that prays, the man that is human, the man that might be just enough like us to show us how it is done. The technology of the Medical Center gave my son more life. One of the great men of the Medical Center gave me the 'Golden Hours' theory that made that time so wondrously valuable. Could anyone convince me that one is less important than the other? I guess that is the crux of what I am trying to say.

I look on the Medical Center with new love and appreciation because I realize more than ever what it all really means. It has returned to me the joy of a child in things new and wondrous and his accept-

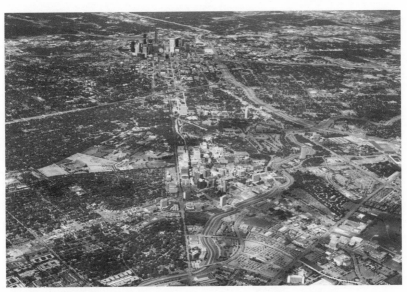

Texas Medical Center, 2002. Courtesy Texas Medical Center

ance of what cannot change. It has given me the ability to find those things to honor above the pangs that would blind me to the good were I not aware that man is a force and his technology is his tool. Even in personal sorrow and that which touches me deeply here, in compassion for others, I can look and find answers in the example before me to help me see the way it really is.

There is more, yet what I have quoted is more than sufficient to justify my earlier remark that these are the only rewards that those who made this Medical Center possible need.

I have finished my reminiscent trip back through time. It has been a memorable one. So much more that happened comes into my mind quite vividly but I have omitted many of these kaleidoscopic views—it is difficult for me not to report them. Yet, though memorable to me, they probably would be boring to others who were not there. I will sit back, relax, and be thankful for all the greatness that has come to this—*our* Texas Medical Center.

EPILOGUE

⁓

IN FREDERICK ELLIOTT'S original manuscript, he wrote a whimsical epilogue in which he contemplated how amazed many of his former colleagues would be if they could come back for a tour of "their" Texas Medical Center. He described the many buildings and noted how much the Medical Center had grown since its beginnings. "In deep reverie I am walking through the Medical Center," he wrote, "stopping now and then in a state of wonderment for all that I see. My mind flashes back to the day that I left the Medical Center offices for the last time. As I continue my stroll on this day in May, 1976, I can hardly believe it . . . even though I've been here and watched it happen."

Elliott's walk began in front of the Jesse H. Jones Library Building, which also housed his Medical Center office. From here, he looked toward the John Freeman Building, the first structure for the University of Texas Health Science Center at Houston Medical School. Elliott then turned his gaze to the north to see additional buildings under construction for the University of Texas Medical School, a large addition underway at Hermann Hospital, and the uniquely designed Martha G. Dunn Memorial Chapel. To the east Elliott could see Ben Taub Hospital, the city-county hospital that had generated so much controversy during his years as executive director of the Medical Center. As he turned to the south, Elliott saw the Methodist Hospital complex, the Texas Woman's University School of Nursing, March Culmore Hall, and the Favrot Building. A little further down Bertner Avenue stood the Institute of Religion. "It rounds out the total purpose for our Medical Center," wrote Elliott. "That is, for the care of all phases of man— religious, mental, and physical."

St. Luke's Hospital, Texas Children's Hospital, and the Texas Heart Institute came into his view as he walked beyond the Methodist Hospital complex. As his gaze turned toward the M. D. Anderson Cancer Center, Elliott reflected upon the generosity of Marshall and Lillie Johnson, who, in 1959, provided a seventeen million dollar gift to the University of Texas for the

Lutheran Pavilion Building, the largest gift ever received by the university up to that time. The building would be officially dedicated on October 1, 1976—nearly twenty years after Marshall Johnson first approached Dr. Elliott to inquire about how to donate money to build a hospital in the Medical Center. Elliott described many other buildings and institutions, including his beloved University of Texas Dental Branch, the Baylor College of Medicine, the Texas Research Institute of Mental Sciences, and The Institute for Rehabilitation and Research, a facility that Elliott recalled Dr. Bertner had wanted in the Medical Center from the beginning. "As I returned to the 'land of now,'" wrote Elliott, "I could not help but reflect upon the rich rewards I have received through the years by having the opportunity to know and be with people like this group who helped to build the Texas Medical Center. In the hearts of many, they will never be forgotten. Time moves on."

I could not help but wonder what Dr. Elliott would say if he could see how the Texas Medical Center has grown in the years since he retired. By the year 2000, the Texas Medical Center had expanded to encompass over seven hundred acres of land, with twenty-two million gross square feet in physical plant space, contained in some one hundred permanent buildings. Over one hundred thousand people visit the Medical Center every day. Twelve miles of private and public streets and roads traverse the Medical Center with fourteen parking garages and twenty-eight surface lots owned and operated by TMC for visitor and staff parking. There are forty-two nonprofit institutions in the Medical Center with combined operating budgets of $4.6 billion. It is estimated that the Medical Center had an indirect impact of some $11.5 billion on the Houston economy. In 2000, the Texas Medical Center recorded 5.4 million patient visits, including 19,307 international patients. As the sixtieth anniversary of the Texas Medical Center approaches in 2005, it has exceeded even the broadest dreams of Bertner, Bates, Elliott, Freeman, Wilkins and the scores of people who contributed in so many ways.

Although Dr. Elliott retired as executive director in 1962, he remained actively involved in the affairs of the Texas Medical Center for the rest of his life in his capacity as a member of the board of trustees. Along with these duties, he wrote this autobiographical manuscript and served as a consultant to the president at the M. D. Anderson Cancer Center and consultant to the University Cancer Foundation.

Among his many other activities, Fred Elliott served on the board of the Marshall and Lillie Johnson Foundation. It seems that he first met the Johnsons sometime during the mid-1950s when Marshall G. Johnson visited Dr. Elliott in his office and announced that he and his wife, Lillie, wished to

TABLE I. *Texas Medical Center Growth, 1963–2000*

	1963	1973	1983	1993	2000
Patient Visits	806, 656	1,252,268	2,200,000	3,087,664	5,446,000
Licensed Beds	2,641	3,486	4,520	6,694	6,014
Students	2,011	5,002	4,520	11,200	16,547
Employees	9,031	17,586	28,633	54,774	61,041

Source: Texas Medical Center Public Affairs

donate funds to build a Lutheran Hospital in the Texas Medical Center. El-liott advised them that they should create a non-profit foundation to handle the business and tax issues involved with making large charitable contribu-tions. During the next few years, Fred Elliott continued to advise the John-sons, and after he retired as executive director of the Texas Medical Center, he joined the board of directors of the Marshall G. and Lillie Johnson Foundation.[1]

Over the years, Fred Elliott and John H. Freeman, one of the original trustees of the M. D. Anderson Foundation, also had become very good friends. When Francis M. Law, Freeman's co-trustee on the board of the Max Krost Charitable Trust, died in 1973, Freeman turned to his trusted old friend, Fred Elliott, to fill the position. The Krost Trust held about a half mil-lion dollars in assets and was originally established in 1945 by the heirs of Max Krost, a wealthy Houston-area grocer, to fund worthy charitable causes. By May, 1973, Fred Elliott found himself on the board of trustees for two chari-table foundations and in a position to direct significant financial support to worthy causes. He quickly discovered a developing program at Texas Lu-theran College (now Texas Lutheran University) in Seguin that enabled him to focus his public health, educational, and humanitarian interests and also provided an opportunity to fulfill one of the dreams of the Medical Center's founders of reaching out into the surrounding communities.

The exact date is lost to history, but evidence suggests that Dr. Elliott first visited the campus of Texas Lutheran College during 1973 in conjunction with his duties as a board member and representative of the Johnson Foun-dation. The Johnsons were Lutherans and very supportive of the college and of other causes and activities of the Lutheran Church. The school had launched a five-year campaign in 1971 to raise four million dollars for building and other operational improvements. The Johnson Foundation contributed $192,400 to the campaign, which helped establish the Johnson Health and Fitness Center in the Jesse H. Jones Physical Education Complex on the campus. Elliott was very impressed with the college during his first trip and again on subsequent visits. The school's fine academic programs and the efforts to blend the spiritual and academic lives of its students with physical fitness and nutrition, the "overall health" concept, struck a chord with Dr. Elliott.[2]

Within months of his first visit to Texas Lutheran College, the school contacted the Krost Charitable Trust, possibly at Elliott's suggestion. The school was interested in creating a full-fledged health maintenance program for students that would function along with the academic program. In 1974, officials at Texas Lutheran submitted a proposal requesting a five thousand dollar grant from the Krost Charitable Trust to fund an initial study for the fitness and nutrition program. The proposal stated, "The Texas Medical Center in Houston is respectfully requested to provide guidance with respect to the program, tests, and the goals of the program. The encouragement we have received from Dr. Elliott and his associates is very important to the faculty and administration of Texas Lutheran College." The Krost Trust awarded this initial grant and provided funding for several additional proposals during the next two years to continue the development of the health and nutrition program.[3]

On September 18, 1976, the new Jesse H. Jones Physical Education Complex at Texas Lutheran College was formally dedicated. Dr. Frederick C. Elliott represented the Johnson Foundation and the Krost Charitable Trust at the ceremonies. In his brief remarks, he observed that the students who attended the school would have the "knowledge and desire to take on . . . the total care of themselves. They will know that their spiritual, mental, and physical self cannot be separated—each 'self' is interrelated to the other in a practical and usable manner. I know the trustees of the Johnson Foundation and the Krost Trust wish the officers and faculty of Texas Lutheran College 'God Speed' in their stewardship of this—a new beginning in developing a whole person for a whole life."[4]

Dr. Elliott had helped to direct considerable financial support from the Johnson Foundation and the Krost Charitable Trust to Texas Lutheran College and had been very generous with his time and energy on behalf of the school. He also proved to be an invaluable connection to the resources of the Texas Medical Center. During spring commencement ceremonies, on May 22, 1977, Texas Lutheran College recognized his efforts and deep commitment by awarding him the degree of Doctor of Humane Letters. This rarely conferred degree was a great honor for Dr. Elliott.[5]

During the next few months, Fred Elliott and John Freeman watched the development of Texas Lutheran's health, fitness, and nutrition program with great interest. By 1977, the Krost Trust had limited assets, limited income, and two trustees who were getting older. John Freeman's eyesight was fading and Fred Elliott's hearing had become so bad that he usually wore powerful hearing aids in both ears. Because of this, the two men concluded that the objectives of the trust would be served best if it was terminated and all assets transferred "to a suitable operating charitable entity." They believed that the "whole health" program that Texas Lutheran College was developing made the school a suitable entity to which the assets could be given. But, the school was in the process of conducting a search for a permanent president. The future of the school's fitness and nutrition programs depended upon who was selected as the school's new leader. The search committee chose Dr. Charles H. Oestreich, who had been the academic dean and acting president, to fill the position on a permanent basis. On the Monday following the announcement, Elliott called Oestreich to inform him that the Krost Charitable Trust was considering a transfer of its remaining assets, some $450,000, to Texas Lutheran College. But, Elliott and Freeman wanted to be assured that the proposed life enrichment program lined up exactly with the expressed intent of the Krost Trust. A team of college administrators led by Dr. Oestreich went to Houston to meet with Elliott and Freeman. Years later, Oestreich recalled that Dr. Elliott "really pressed" the Texas Lutheran College administration "in a positive way" to ensure that the Krost Life Enrichment Program clearly met all provisions and requirements as defined by the Krost Trust. Elliott strongly believed in preventive medicine and saw this program as an opportunity to instill in young people the good health habits that would enable them to lead vigorous, productive lives.[6]

Finally, on October 31, 1977, during a luncheon to commemorate Dr. Charles H. Oestreich's inauguration as president of Texas Lutheran College, Dr. Elliott formally announced that all of the assets of the Max Krost Charitable Trust, worth nearly $450,000, would be transferred to the school. The funds would be used to finance the new Health Fitness and Nutrition Program designed "to help students and others establish a pattern of living that will be conducive to good mental, spiritual and physical health." Elliott's vision of improved public health through preventive medicine and education now had a place to take root and grow on the campus of Texas Lutheran College.[7]

The following year, Texas Lutheran administrators floated the idea of creating an endowed chair to honor Fred Elliott's contributions to the college. Dr. Elliott had played an instrumental role as a facilitator and benefactor, and the university convinced the Johnson Foundation to donate the funds to establish the endowment. In December, 1978, the Johnson Foundation gave $500,000 to endow the Frederick C. Elliott Chair in Health Fitness and Nutrition. Lillie Johnson added an additional gift to help establish the chair.[8] This would be the capstone of a distinguished career that spanned nearly seventy years in which he served as a pharmacist, dentist, educator, administrator, public health advocate, co-founder of the Texas Medical Center and foundation trustee. Elliott received many letters, telegrams, and messages of congratulations from colleagues and friends across the state. The endowed chair would be a "living" testimony to a lifetime of service in health care and an appropriate tribute to a man who believed strongly in the importance of education.[9]

The years that followed Frederick Elliott's retirement as executive director of the Texas Medical Center at age sixty-nine had been some of the most fruitful but also some of the most difficult of his life. Apart from his continuing professional and humanitarian endeavors, it appears that during the early years of his retirement, Fred and Ann Elliott enjoyed touring the country in their travel trailer.

Eventually, they sold the trailer and their house on Quenby Street near Rice University and moved from Houston to the scenic town of Kerrville, which is located in the Texas Hill Country northwest of San Antonio. For a few years, while he was heavily involved with the Krost Trust and the M. D. Anderson Cancer Center, the Elliotts moved back to an apartment in Houston. But, sometime during 1979 or early in 1980, Fred and Ann Elliott again packed their belongings and moved to a mobile home court in the more affordable town of Kerrville.

At the time of his retirement in 1962, Dr. Elliott confessed that he had not managed his money with an eye toward his retirement years and pension programs were just becoming a major component of professional employment packages. Although he did not have a pension package, the Texas Medical Center had deferred some of his earnings and created a plan to pay him $300 per month for 198 months (16.5 years) after he retired. By 1979, Fred Elliott essentially had outlived his "retirement" and his deferred income funds were nearly exhausted. He may have been eligible for social security, but had no other pension available to him.[10]

Fred Elliott was a proud man and would not accept charity from anyone.

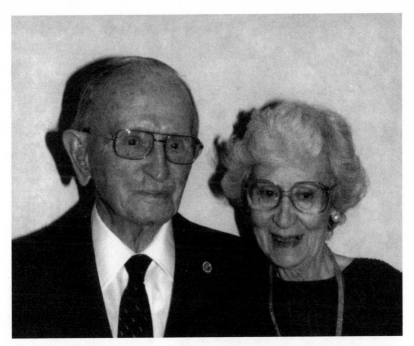

Last known photograph of Ann and Fred Elliott together, taken a few months before his death in 1986.

But his friends, former colleagues, and students at the University of Texas Dental Branch occasionally provided an honorarium for him. During the mid-1970s, Elliott's good friend, Dr. R. Lee Clark, president of the M. D. Anderson Cancer Institute, offered Elliott a part-time appointment as consultant to the president. His duties included "collaboration with Don Macon in the preparation of historical information concerning M. D. Anderson and other University of Texas institutions in the Texas Medical Center." Elliott served in this capacity from June 1, 1975, until August 8, 1977, when for unknown reasons, Elliott and Lee Clark agreed to end the appointment. Dr. Elliott continued in an unpaid capacity as a consultant to the president.[11]

By late 1986, at age ninety-three, Fred Elliott's health was failing. He had developed heart disease and needed more care than Ann could provide for him at home. He was admitted to the Hilltop Village Nursing Home in Kerrville where he died of a stroke on New Year's Eve, December 31, 1986. A memorial service was held on January 14, 1987, in the auditorium of the Uni-

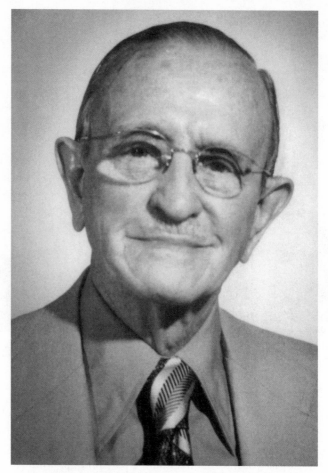

Dr. Frederick C. Elliott in 1986. Courtesy E. W. D'Anton

versity of Texas Dental Branch in the Texas Medical Center. The list of speakers who eulogized Dr. Elliott included John V. Olson, D.D.S., Dean Emeritus of the University of Texas Health Science Center at Houston Dental Branch; Richard E. Wainerdi, Ph.D., President of the Texas Medical Center; and David M. Mumford, M.D., Associate Dean and Director, Office of Continuing Education, Baylor College of Medicine. The Rev. Julian Byrd, Director of Pastoral Care and Education at Hermann Hospital, gave the invocation and benediction. Elliott was remembered as one of the nine signers of the original charter of incorporation for the Texas Medical Center. He was lauded as "a visionary with a practical turn of mind that made his visions come true" and as "a planter and later shepherd of all we see around us today—the awesome yet still awakening Texas Medical Center." Richard E. Wainerdi said, "I think the most impressive way to remember Dr. Elliott is to look around you. When you look around and see the Texas Medical Center, that is Dr. Elliott's monument. It is, in fact, his legacy."[12]

The legacy of Frederick Chesley Elliott continues on the grounds of the Texas Medical Center and on the campus of Texas Lutheran University. Fred Elliott was a man of vision, determination, and compassion who cared deeply about public health, about education, and about the Texas Medical Center. Tragedy visited him at an early age, but Elliott learned the hard lessons of his youth. These lessons forged him into the kind of man who could withstand the political storms and administrative pressures that often swirled around him as an adult. Elliott was an innovator, an original thinker who dared to look into the future and tried to shape it for the betterment of humanity.

Elliott saw his role as both a responsibility and an opportunity to speak out for improved public health in Houston. He was the first to take the idea of a center for health education so far as to commission an architect's drawing of a proposed building and even constructed miniature plaster models to help publicize the idea. His friendship with men like Dr. E. W. Bertner, William B. Bates, John H. Freeman, and other community leaders played a role in the development of a great medical center for Houston. Each contributed their ideas and energy, publicly supported the concept, and worked long and hard to ensure a first-class medical facility.

As executive director of the Texas Medical Center (the title evolved over the years from director, to executive director, to president), Dr. Elliott worked closely with the board of directors to encourage philanthropists to support its institutions and to provide funds for new facilities. He grappled with many of the same problems that plague Texas Medical Center leaders today including rapid growth, traffic congestion, limited parking and the frequent flooding caused by the tropical rains that often inundate the city. Elliott's calm demeanor and willingness to work behind the scenes earned the respect of many contemporaries. When he announced his retirement in 1962, famed attorney Leon Jaworski wrote to him saying, "I am one of those who happens to have some information on how valuable you have been to the Center from the very beginning, and I look forward with much anticipation to continuing to work with you in the furtherance of this great cause." Houston businessman and investor, Laurence H. Favrot wrote, "May I take this occasion to express to you my personal esteem and the great respect with which you are held by all who are familiar with your dedicated work to the Texas Medical Center during its important formative years." And Aris A. Mallas, Jr., project director of the Austin-based Texas Research League, wrote to Medical Center board member Hines H. Baker, "Dr. Elliott is an outstanding [executive] director of the Center, but of even greater importance to this State, he is the only person in the state knowledgeable in medical planning who has the respect and confidence of our Texas Legislature. Dr. Elliott is thought of as not only being competent, but impartial as well." Mallas stated that Elliott's retirement might leave "a deep void that it may take years to fill."[13]

In 1999, the Texas Medical Center published a master plan to guide and coordinate future growth. Within one year, it became apparent that the Medical Center was growing faster than what had been anticipated in the master plan. Dr. Elliott's legacy, the Texas Medical Center, continues to thrive to an extent that would surprise even him.

Former First Lady Barbara Bush once called the Texas Medical Center "Houston's gift to the world." "This is the largest and most successful medical center in the history of the world," said Richard Wainerdi, "There are very few places in the world where this much good is done." Although he has not yet received the public recognition that he deserves for all of his efforts on behalf of "Houston's gift to the world," there is no doubt that Fred Elliott accomplished much that was good during his lifetime. The impact of his life's work will be felt by millions of people for decades to come.[14]

NOTES

~

INTRODUCTION

1. Mavis P. Kelsey, Sr., *Twentieth-Century Doctor: House Calls to Space Medicine* (College Station: Texas A&M University Press, 1999) 189–91. *See also* Mavis P. Kelsey, Sr., *Doctoring in Houston* (Houston: Kelsey-Seybold Foundation, 1996) 10–11.

2. *1970 Annual Report of the Texas Medical Center, Inc.,* 92.

3. N. Don Macon, *Mr. John H. Freeman and Friends: A Story of the Texas Medical Center and How It Began* (Houston: Texas Medical Center, 1973) 33.

4. N. Don Macon, *South From Flower Mountain: A Conversation with William B. Bates* (Houston: Texas Medical Center, 1975) 65. Col. William B. Bates (honorary title) was born on August 16, 1889, near Nacogdoches, Texas, one of thirteen children. He taught school and later attended the University of Texas Law School in Austin. Bates graduated in 1915, first in his class. He served in the army during World War I and was twice wounded during action in France. After the war, he went into law practice with his brother and was elected district attorney of Nacogdoches County. He later moved to Houston and joined the firm of Fulbright and Crooker on January 1, 1923. He became a partner in Fulbright, Crooker, Freeman and Bates on January 1, 1928. Bates handled some of the legal work for Anderson Clayton & Company and became good friends with and a fishing companion of Monroe D. Anderson.

5. *Papers of Frederick C. Elliott, D.D.S.,* Manuscript Collection No. 71 of the Harris County Medical Archive, Houston Academy of Medicine–Texas Medical Center Library (HAM–TMC Library), McGovern Historical Collections and Research Center.

6. N. Don Macon, *Monroe Dunaway Anderson, His Legacy: A History of the Texas Medical Center, 50ᵗʰ Anniversary Edition* (Houston: Texas Medical Center, 1994) 64–65; Macon, *John H. Freeman,* 19. The law firm exists today as Fulbright & Jaworski.

7. Frederick C. Elliott, interview by William D. Seybold, August 9, 1971.

8. Don E. Carleton, *A Breed So Rare: The Life of J. R. Parten, Liberal Texas Oil Man, 1896–1992* (Austin: Texas State Historical Association, 1998) 140–43. For more on William Pitt Ballinger see John Anthony Moretta, *William Pitt*

Ballinger: Texas Lawyer, Southern Statesman, 1825–1888 (Austin: Texas State Historical Association, 2000).

9. Carleton, *A Breed So Rare,* 206–209; Chester Burns, interview by William H. Kellar, July 16, 2001.

10. Ibid., 207; Chester Burns, interview by William H. Kellar, July 16, 2001.

11. *The University of Texas Medical Branch at Galveston: A Seventy-five Year History by the Faculty and Staff* (Austin: University of Texas Press, 1967) 163; Chester Burns, interview by William H. Kellar, July 16, 2001; Carlton, *A Breed So Rare,* 208–209.

12. Carleton, *A Breed So Rare,* 207–209; Chester Burns, interview by William H. Kellar, July 16, 2001. *See also* Chester R. Burns, *Saving Lives, Training Caregivers, Making Discoveries: A Centennial History of the University of Texas Medical Branch at Galveston* (Austin: Texas State Historical Association, 2003) 46–54.

13. Frederick C. Elliott, interview by William D. Seybold, August 9, 1971. *See also* Marilyn McAdams Sibley, *The Methodist Hospital of Houston: Serving the World* (Austin: Texas State Historical Association, 1989) 102–103. Sibley notes: "Early in the twentieth century, many Galveston businesses moved inland to Houston, and by 1941 the Anderson trustees and other interested parties thought the time had come for the Medical Branch to follow suit."

14. Carleton, *A Breed So Rare,* 227–33; *The University of Texas Medical Branch at Galveston,* 163–67; Chester Burns, interview by William H. Kellar, July 16, 2001.

15. Thomas D. Anderson, interview by William H. Kellar, January 26, 2000; Macon, *South From Flower Mountain,* 62; Macon, *John H. Freeman,* 21–22.

16. Chester Burns, interview by William H. Kellar, July 16, 2001; Carleton, *A Breed So Rare,* 226–33; *The University of Texas Medical Branch at Galveston,* 163.

17. *The University of Texas Medical Branch at Galveston,* 164–68; Chester Burns, interview by William H. Kellar, July 16, 2001.

18. R. W. Cumley and Joan McCay, eds., *The First Twenty Years of the University of Texas M. D. Anderson Hospital and Tumor Institute* (Houston: University of Texas M. D. Anderson Hospital and Tumor Institute, 1964) 23. The University of Texas Board of Regents agreed to call the cancer hospital the M. D. Anderson Hospital for Cancer Research of the University of Texas on September 25, 1942. Over the years, the cancer center has had several name changes and is known today as the University of Texas M. D. Anderson Cancer Center.

19. Clyde W. Burleson and Suzy Williams Burleson, *A Guide to the Texas Medical Center* (Austin: University of Texas Press, 1987) 2; Macon, *Monroe Dunaway Anderson,* 103.

20. Cumley and McCay, eds., *The First Twenty Years,* 1–9. By 1937, Congress had created the National Cancer Institute as a part of the U.S. Public Health Service. With more than 400,000 cases of cancer reported, the disease had become second only to heart disease as the leading cause of death in the United States.

21. Ibid., 11.

22. Ibid., 13; Frederick C. Elliott, interview by William D. Seybold, August 9, 1971; Macon, *John H. Freeman*, 25–27.

23. Cumley and McCay, eds., *The First Twenty Years*, 5–17; Macon, *John H. Freeman*, 26.

24. Macon, *John H. Freeman*, 25.

25. Cumley and McCay, eds., *The First Twenty Years*, 19–22. The Anderson Foundation acquired "The Oaks" estate of Capt. James Baker in Houston during the summer of 1942. The estate became the temporary home of the cancer hospital until the permanent facility opened in the Texas Medical Center in 1954. Ernst W. Bertner was named as the acting director of the hospital until R. Lee Clark was appointed permanent director in 1946.

26. Macon, *John H. Freeman*, 27; William B. Bates, "History and Development of the Texas Medical Center," speech to Texas Gulf Coast Historical Association, November 20, 1956. Transcript courtesy Richard E. Wainerdi, TMC president.

27. E. W. D'Anton, *Memories: A History of the University of Texas Dental Banch at Houston* (Houston: University of Texas Health Science Center at Houston Dental Branch, 1991) 20–22; Macon, *John H. Freeman*, 28; E. W. Bertner, "Commencement Address to UT School of Dentistry Class, June 10, 1946," E. W. Bertner Speeches and Medical Papers File, Bertner Notebooks, Manuscript Collection of the Harris County Medical Archive, HAM–TMC Library, McGovern Historical Collections and Research Center.

28. Burleson and Burleson, *A Guide to the Texas Medical Center*, 3; Macon, *John H. Freeman*, 28; Macon, *Monroe Dunaway Anderson*, 88–92, 102–103; Richard E. Wainerdi, "Texas Medical Center," address to the Newcomen Society of the United States, November 19, 1992, Houston; Thomas D. Anderson, interview by William H. Kellar, January 26, 2000. W. Leland Anderson and Thomas D. Anderson are the nephews of Monroe D. Anderson.

29. Macon, *John H. Freeman*, 36.

30. Denton A. Cooley, interview by William H. Kellar, December 26, 2000; Mavis P. Kelsey, Sr., interview by William H. Kellar, September 19, 2000.

CHAPTER I

1. The flu pandemic of 1918–19 killed 675,000 Americans. In Philadelphia, nearly eleven thousand people died within the first month after the flu arrived in the fall of 1918. During October, 1918, 200,000 died in the United States. Worldwide, estimates of the number of people who perished from the virus range from twenty million to as many as one hundred million. The 1918 flu was "twenty-five times more deadly than ordinary influenza." The illness struck quickly, causing severe hemorrhaging that often caused the patient to die within hours of the first symptoms. Curiously, it tended to afflict healthy young people

rather than the elderly, the very young, or the infirm. *See* Gina Kolata, *Flu: The Story of the Great Influenza Pandemic of 1918 and the Search for the Virus That Caused It* (New York: Touchstone, 1999) 6–20.

2. *Calender of Events, Frederick Chesley Elliott, Ph.D., D.D.S.,* Elliott Papers. The child, a boy, was named Frederick C. Elliott, Jr.

3. Elliott's second wife, Phrania Anna Orr, was born in St. Joseph, Mo., to Josephe Hyram Orr and Samantha Lurilla Thomas Conley Orr on May 28, 1905.

CHAPTER 2

1. Elliott wrote: "One hundred years later, in 1940, I was a guest of the American Dental Association and the Maryland State Dental Association. I had been invited to be a guest lecturer on the program for the 'Centenary of Dentistry,' commemorating the opening of the Baltimore College of Dentistry. Many dentists who practiced in Texas were graduates of this college. I should mention briefly that nineteen years later, May 16, 1959, I was honored by receiving the 'Dentist of the Century' award of the American Dental Association from the Houston District Dental Society. The dental college in Baltimore was this much older than the American Dental Association."

2. *See* D'Anton, *Memories,* 2–4.

3. Elliott wrote: "He [Dr. M. S. Merchant] took part in the activities of many dental organizations. In August of 1904, he attended a meeting of the Fourth International Dental Congress of the Federation Dentaire Internationale. This congress met in the United States at the time of the St. Louis World's Fair. Dr. Harvey Burkhardt was chairman of the Congress. I mention him because of his many contributions to dentistry. Later I became acquainted with Dr. Burkhardt. I had met him at some of my early lectures to dental societies. Thirty-one years later, in the fall of 1935, I became a member of the Federation Dentaire Internationale. I lectured at the Ninth International Dental Congress in Vienna, Austria, in August, 1936."

4. Elliott wrote: "It is important that I name these appointees since they were not only members of the first faculty of the dental college, but also they were instrumental in preserving the integrity of the college through many trying years. Dr. O. F. Gambati was elected dean of the college. The following members were elected professors: (Note the number of subjects each was to teach!) O. F. Gambati, D.D.S., Professor of Dental Histology, Dental Anatomy and Orthodontia; Thomas P. Williams, D.D.S., Professor of Operative Dentistry, Dental Surgery, and Oral Hygiene; Charles H. Edge (preceptor trained), Professor of Dental Pathology; Dental Materia Medica and Therapeutics and Crown and Bridge Work; M. J. Lossing, D.D.S., Professor of Prosthetic Dentistry and Dental Metallurgy; R. T. Morris, M.D., Professor of Anatomy and Materia

Medica and Therapeutics; E. M. Armstrong, M.D., A.B., A.M., Professor of Physiology, Oral Surgery, Hygiene; W. A. Haley, M.D., Professor of Histology, Pathology, and Bacteriology; and P. S. Tilson, M.Sc., Professor of Chemistry. The following members of the faculty were elected as lecturers, instructors, or demonstrators: C. A. Lee, Lecturer and Clinical Instructor in Porcelain Art; C. S. Preston, D.D.S., Instructor in Crown and Bridge Work; W. H. Scherer, D.D.S., Instructor and Demonstrator in Prosthetic Dentistry and Dental Metallurgy; H. T. Hamblin, D.D.S., Instructor in Dental Technique; W. N. Shaw, M.D., Demonstrator of Anatomy; W. G. Priester, M.D., Demonstrator of Bacteriology and Histology; A. T. Hunt, Ph.D., Instructor in Pharmacy; Ed S. Phelps, Lecturer on Dental Jurisprudence."

5. Ralph C. Cooley was the father of Denton A. Cooley, who performed the first successful heart transplant in the United States in 1968.

6. Walter Cronkite, Jr., later went on to become a nationally famous TV journalist at CBS.

CHAPTER 3

1. See introduction of the book for detailed account of Dr. Spies's role.

2. Cumley and McCay, eds., *The First Twenty Years*, 13–17.

3. *See* Macon, *Monroe Dunaway Anderson.*

4. Elliott wrote: "In 1918, all of us in the senior class at the Kansas City Dental College realized that the news that we read at the time made it clear that we would be called into service. We must report immediately to the Army Induction Center for a physical examination and be inducted into the Army. When would we leave? What would happen to the school? We were tremendously relieved when after a few days we were informed that we were privates in the Medical Enlisted Reserve Corp (MERC) of the United States Army. We would not be called to active duty until we had completed our education. This applied to all classes."

5. Chauncey D. Leake became vice president for medical affairs of the University of Texas in September, 1942. A special committee of faculty members at the Medical Branch was appointed by the board of regents to recommend a vice president for the Medical Branch. Among the members of this committee were Judson Taylor (member of the board of trustees of the Texas Dental College and president of the Texas State Medical Association) and Cabe Terrell of Fort Worth, president of the University of Texas Alumni Association. They recommended Dr. Leake for the position.

6. *See* Cumley and McCay, eds., *The First Twenty Years*, 25–26. The authors note that "although the Baker Estate was a most welcome endowment," it also brought several unique and unwelcome problems for a cancer research institution. "There were the rats, the big, gray wood rats that infested the place.

Mr. Smith, the night watchman, waged a continuing battle against the rats. He would shoot at them with his .38 Smith and Wesson, but often instead of hitting the rat he would hit a steam pipe under which the rat had dived." The stable–carriage house was converted to laboratory space, but the facility was inhabited by pigeons and with pigeons came fleas, which "spread everywhere, throughout the laboratories, in clothes, in hair. The biochemists were plagued by them."

7. *See* D'Anton, *Memories*, 20–23.

8. Cumley and McCay, eds., *The First Twenty Years*, 28.

CHAPTER 4

1. Oveta Culp Hobby was the wife of former Texas governor William P. Hobby, Sr., and served as the first commander of the Women's Army Corps and first secretary of the Department of Health, Education, and Welfare (1953–55). The Hobby family was very successful in newspaper publishing, television, and radio in Houston. Hugh Roy Cullen was a wealthy oilman and philanthropist. In 1947, he established the Cullen Foundation to support education and medicine. Jesse H. Jones was a successful Houston businessman, newspaper publisher, New Deal official, and secretary of commerce during Franklin D. Roosevelt's third term. Because of his philanthropy and community leadership, he was also known as "Mr. Houston."

2. *Houston Post*, March 1, 1946. George A. Hill's grandfather had fought in the Battle of San Jacinto where Texas won independence from Mexico in 1836. Hill was president of the Houston Oil Company and was known for his philanthropy and community leadership.

3. Elliott wrote: "I presented this plan to the board in 1962 at the time that I informed them that I had plans to retire as executive director. I suggested that the plan be started at that time. Also, I mentioned that I would like to continue with the Medical Center as the development officer if the plan was approved. The trustees were aware that I had been performing the duties of both a development officer and the director of the Medical Center. I suggested that these two duties be separated so that the executive officer of the Medical Center could be relieved of the responsibility of development activities that I had been doing. Also I believed that it was important for the Medical Center to take a more active part in the procurement of funds. The development officer would assist in the procurement of funds that were needed by the institutions in the Medical Center for their expanded programs, for endowment of chairs, and other needed permanently supported projects. I pointed out that it would not be too difficult to convince the officers of the present foundations on the need to consult with the development office before considering grant requests from the institutions in the Medical Center. This action would allow the trustees of the Medical Center to learn of the proposed expansions that the institutions had

planned before they had been funded. The trustees would not be in the position of being called upon to deed land for programs that they had not officially approved. These suggestions were made in support of my recommendations for establishing an office for development. Then I explained to the trustees how the office would operate. The director was to report to the board of trustees when requested to do so by the president of the Texas Medical Center. The director of development would keep the executive officer of the Medical Center informed of his actions and would follow suggestions from him for programs for which he needed funds. The development plan was approved by the board and I was appointed as director of development on a half-time basis. Later this plan was changed by the board of trustees. The development plan was to be a function of the executive office. However, I remained with the Medical Center until the first part of 1963, at which time I resigned."

4. *Houston Post,* May 11, 1946.

5. *Houston Post,* July 17, 1946.

6. *Houston Post,* July 13, 15, 18, 19, 1946. Randolph Lee Clark, Jr., was born July 2, 1906, in the Texas Panhandle town of Hereford. He earned his medical degree at the Medical College of Virginia, interned at Garfield Memorial Hospital in Washington, D.C., and was selected for a residency at the American Hospital in Paris, France, where he also continued his studies at the University of Paris Medical School. Following this, Clark spent the next five years in Minnesota at the Mayo Foundation for Medical Education and Research, where he specialized in general surgery and cancer surgery. During World War II, Clark enlisted in the Army Air Corps Medical Department. Prior to his appointment to the M. D. Anderson Hospital and Tumor Institute, he was stationed at Randolph Field in San Antonio, where he was the director of surgical research and the department of surgery at the School of Aviation Medicine.

7. *Houston Post,* June 2, 1946.

8. *Houston Post,* September 4, 1946.

9. Sibley, *The Methodist Hospital of Houston,* 75–78.

10. *Houston Post,* June 23, 1946.

11. *Houston Post,* January 11, 1947.

12. *Houston Post,* March 25, 1947.

13. *Houston Post,* March 10, 1947; Elliott wrote: "It is worthy that I note here that as I was writing the preceding few lines about Mr. Hughes, on April 6, 1976, I was told that Mr. Hughes had died in a private plane just ready to make a landing at the Houston International Airport. He was being brought to the Medical Center in his hometown (for which he had not contributed any of his great wealth), but he did not make it."

14. *Houston Post,* March 28, 29, 1947.

15. *Houston Chronicle,* December 19, 1947, January 7, 8, 20, 1948; *Houston Post,* January 19, 1948; *Houston Press,* January 7, 19, 1948.

16. *Houston Post,* June 27, 1948.

17. *Houston Post,* April 4, 24, 1948.
18. *Houston Post,* July 22, 23, 1948.
19. Denton A. Cooley, interview by William H. Kellar, December 26, 2000; Michael DeBakey, interview by William H. Kellar, January 25, 2001.

CHAPTER 5

1. *Houston Post,* May 12, 1949.
2. Elliott also stated: "One might recall that it was in 1974 that President Nixon had ordered that the Marine Hospital in Galveston be closed. This action had been recommended to President Nixon because for some time the Marine Hospital had operated with less than 50 percent of the hospital beds in use. Pressure from Galveston groups caused President Nixon to rescind his action. I cannot help but remark that had this been a private hospital, it would have been closed long before President Nixon's action. Everyone wants taxes reduced just so tax reductions do not effect their 'pet projects.'"
3. R. Lee Clark and R. W. Cumley, eds. *The Book of Health* (Houston: Elsevier Press, Inc., 1953). Cumley and Clark collaborated on the massive tome.
4. Sibley, *The Methodist Hospital of Houston,* 10–12, 92.
5. Elliott wrote: "In 1976 we realized that no one would have predicted how right we were, but how far wrong we were in our estimate of the increase."
6. J. Searcy Bracewell, Jr., interview by William H. Kellar, October 4, 2000. Searcy Bracewell, a Houston attorney, represented Harris County (Houston) in the Texas State Legislature during the early years of the Texas Medical Center.
7. Sibley, *The Methodist Hospital of Houston,* 92.
8. *Houston Chronicle,* July 29, 1950; *Houston Post,* July 29, 1950.
9. *The University of Texas Medical Branch at Galveston,* 67–69.

CHAPTER 6

1. *Houston Chronicle,* January 26, 1951.
2. *Houston Chronicle,* May 23, 1951.
3. *Houston Chronicle,* September 23, 1951.
4. *Houston Post,* February 1, 1952; March 26, 1952. Elliott wrote: "At the same meeting of the board of regents on March 26, the bids for the new Dental Branch building were opened. The contract was not awarded this time because the low bid could not be determined. At the time the bids were called many alternate bids were allowed to be made on some of the sub–contracts which accounted for the delay. The award was made later to the Manhattan Construction Company of Houston."
5. *Houston Chronicle,* May 4, 7, and 8, 1952; D'Anton, *Memories,* 26–27.
6. Mavis P. Kelsey, Sr., who trained at the Mayo Clinic, first arrived in Houston in January, 1949. He began a medical practice that eventually became the

Kelsey-Seybold Clinic, a pioneering multispecialty medical clinic. *See* William Henry Kellar and Vaishali J. Patel, *Kelsey- Seybold Clinic: A Legacy of Excellence in Health Care* (Houston: KS Management Services, LLP, 1999); Kelsey, *Twentieth-Century Doctor.*

7. The two students were Moritz Virano Craven, age 24, and Zeb Ferdinand Poindexter, age 23. Craven's father, Essex S. Craven, was a practicing physician, and Poindexter was the son of a school teacher. Craven had a bachelor's degree from Dillard College and a master's degree in education from Texas Southern University. Poindexter earned a bachelor's degree at Wiley College and a master of science degree at Texas Southern University. No comparable dental school existed in Texas for African American students during the Jim Crow era. Craven and Poindexter passed competitive exams and a dental aptitude test established by the American Dental Association before being admitted to the University of Texas Dental Branch. *Houston Post,* September 3, 1952.

8. *Houston Chronicle,* October 1, 1952; *Houston Post,* October 1, 1952; *Houston Press,* October 1, 1952.

9. *Houston Chronicle,* October 16, 1952; *Houston Post,* October 16, 1952; *Houston Press,* October 16, 1952.

10. *See also* Sibley, *The Methodist Hospital of Houston,* 133–34.

11. The new city-county hospital, Ben Taub Hospital, finally opened in the Texas Medical Center on May 16, 1963. Dr. Elliott discusses the controversy surrounding the hospital throughout the book.

12. The *Houston Press* reported on July 30, 1953, that Frederick C. Elliott was "dangerously ill." The brief article noted that Dr. Elliott had a "kidney ailment" and was in Memorial Hospital, where he had undergone "some surgery, but not too extreme." It is typical of Elliott's stoic style not to elaborate on his own illness and suffering.

13. Cumley and Clark's *The Book of Health* can be found at HAM–TMC Library, McGovern Historical Collections and Research Center.

14. The Howard Hughes Medical Institute (HHMI) was chartered in Delaware on December 17, 1953. In 1993, the institute moved to its current headquarters in Chevy Chase, Maryland. During the first fifty years of its existence, the HHMI became an important supporter of improvements in science education in the United States and of biomedical research at more than seventy universities and research centers worldwide. The institute is a nonprofit medical research establishment that employs hundreds of leading biomedical scientists who continue to work at their host institutions. Graduate and medical students and researchers at the University of Texas at Austin, the University of Texas Medical Branch at Galveston, Baylor College of Medicine, and Rice University are among the recent Texas recipients of the HHMI fellowships.

15. *Kansas City Times,* March 8, 1954.

16. *See* Cumley and McCay, eds., *The First Twenty Years,* 74–89.

17. *Houston Post,* August 1, 1954.

18. *Houston Post,* August 22, 1954.

19. *Houston Chronicle,* September 10, 1954; *Houston Post,* September 10, 1954.

20. *Houston Press,* November 29, 1954; Ed Kilman and Theon Wright, *Hugh Roy Cullen: A Story of American Opportunity* (New York: Prentice-Hall, 1954).

21. *Houston Post,* January 30, 1955.

22. *Houston Chronicle,* November 27, December 1, 4, 1955; *Houston Post,* November 30, December 1, 2, 1955.

CHAPTER 7

1. *Houston Post,* April 13, 1956.

2. *Houston Post,* September 27, 1956.

3. *Houston Post,* March 3, 4, 1957.

4. *Houston Post,* May 29, 1958.

5. *Houston Press,* July 11, 1958; *Houston Post,* July 12, 1958. James Anderson had five brothers: Thomas D. Anderson, Ben M. Anderson, Frank C. Anderson, Robert S. Anderson, and W. Leland Anderson.

6. *Houston Post,* July 24, 1958. *See also Houston Press,* July 18, 1958.

7. The Good Samaritan building was announced on January 18, 1959. The story and an architect's rendition of the building appeared in the *Houston Chronicle* on that date. In 2002, the John P. McGovern Commons Building opened in the Texas Medical Center. It has many of the features that Dr. Elliott describes.

8. *Houston Post,* March 13, 1959.

9. *Houston Chronicle,* April 3, 4, 1959; *Houston Post,* April 3, 4, 1959.

10. *Houston Post,* April 4, 1959.

11. *Houston Chronicle,* May 17, 1959; *Houston Post,* May 17, 1959.

12. *Houston Post,* October 13, 1959.

13. *Houston Chronicle,* November 5, 1959; *Houston Post,* November 1, 1959.

14. *Houston Chronicle,* December 4, 1959; *Houston Post,* December 4, 9, 1959.

15. *Houston Chronicle,* December 17, 1959.

16. *Houston Post,* December 31, 1959.

CHAPTER 8

1. Jonas Salk began his research to develop a vaccine against polio in 1947 at the University of Pittsburgh Medical School. On April 12, 1955, he announced that he had completed successful human trials of a vaccine that was composed of "killed" polio virus that was injected and would immunize without the risk of infecting the patient. Albert B. Sabin, at the University of Cincinnati College of Medicine, began human trials of his oral vaccine in 1955. In 1960, his vaccine was used to immunize approximately one hundred million children in Europe.

Vaccinations began in the United States on a large scale in 1962. The Sabin and Salk vaccines have nearly eradicated polio.

2. *Houston Chronicle*, January 3, 1960; *Houston Post*, January 3, 1960.
3. *Houston Chronicle*, February 18, 19, 1960.
4. *Houston Post*, February 15, 1960.
5. *Houston Chronicle*, February 27, 1960; *Houston Post*, February 27, 1960.
6. *Houston Chronicle*, April 27, 1960.
7. *Houston Post*, May 22, 1960.
8. *Houston Chronicle*, May 22, 1960.
9. *Houston Chronicle*, June 2, 1960; Sibley, *The Methodist Hospital of Houston*, 149.
10. *Houston Press*, June 3, 1960; *Houston Chronicle*, June 6, 1960.
11. *Houston Chronicle*, June 6, 1960.
12. *Houston Chronicle*, August 25, 1960.
13. *Houston Chronicle*, October 2, 1960.
14. *Houston Chronicle*, October 30, 1960; Cumley and McCay, eds., *The First Twenty Years*, 184. A. Clark Griffin had found dietary factors that influenced the process of a certain type of liver cancer in rats. In collaboration with a Japanese scientist, he was able to isolate and purify a substance that was only present in cancer tissue. Griffin was to be relieved of most of his administrative duties to devote more time to his research work.

EPILOGUE

1. *Houston Post*, April 4, 1959. The Johnsons' donation was announced anonymously in 1959.
2. *Houston Chronicle*, September 19, 1976. The Houston Endowment, a foundation created by Mr. and Mrs. Jesse H. Jones of Houston, contributed $820,000. The L. E. Mabee Foundation of Tulsa, Okla., put up $100,000 dollars to help fund the Mabee Aquatic Center that also was located in the Jones Physical Education Complex.
3. "Krost Trust Planning Project: The Health Maintenance Program at Texas Lutheran College," Elliott Papers. The school was in the process of developing a life enrichment program and had turned to the Texas Medical Center for help. In a letter to Dr. Elliott in April, 1974, Grant Taylor, then the dean of the University of Texas Health Science Center at Houston, Division of Continuing Education, told Elliott he was "pleased to meet with the group from Seguin and was impressed with the scope of their educational interests." Taylor suggested several "modest projects between the Texas Medical Center and the Seguin Center." He also indicated that "one or more of the above programs might best be initiated through a TMC Biomedical Chair to be established in existing facilities on the Seguin campus." Grant Taylor to Frederick C. Elliott, April 3, 1974.

4. Frederick C. Elliott, "A Magnificent Beginning," remarks at the dedication of the Jesse H. Jones Physical Education Complex at Texas Lutheran College, September 18, 1976.

5. Frederick C. Elliott to C. H. Oestreich, May 6, 1977; *Texas Medical Center News,* February, 1987.

6. Charles Oestreich, interview by William H. Kellar, February 24, 2003. On June 25, 1976, Elliott wrote to Charles H. Oestreich, who at the time was still the acting president of Texas Lutheran College. He told Oestreich that he and John Freeman were "quite pleased with the progress that you have made since the first grant was made to you from the Max Krost Charitable Trust." Frederick C. Elliott to C. H. Oestreich, June 25, 1976.

7. Texas Lutheran College *Torch,* November, 1977; *Lone Star Lutheran,* November 4, 1977. The Krost Life Enrichment Program was designed to "promote a whole person approach to life which integrates the intellectual, spiritual, physical and social well-being of an individual." All Texas Lutheran students are encouraged to enroll in the program. The Krost Program offers internship and work-study programs for students in biology and kinesiology, sponsors an annual symposium, purchases student art, and sponsors other activities.

8. *Texas Medical Center News,* February, 1987; William G. Squires, Jr., interview by William H. Kellar, July 25, 2002.

9. In May, 1980, Texas Lutheran College appointed William G. Squires, Jr., as the first director of the Krost Life Enrichment Program. Squires earned his Ph.D. at Texas A&M University and is presently professor of biology, professor of kinesiology, director of the Krost Life Enrichment Program, and holds the Elliot Chair in Health, Fitness, and Nutrition.

10. W. Leland Anderson to Frederick C. Elliott, April 4, 1957; W. Leland Anderson, memorandum: "Proposed Renewal of Employment contract for Dr. Frederick C. Elliott, June 3, 1959.

11. R. Lee Clark to Frederick C. Elliott, May 26, 1975.

12. Kerr County Bureau of Vital Statistics, Kerrville, Tex.; *Houston Post,* January 9, 1987; *Houston Chronicle,* January 11, 1987; *Texas Medical Center News,* February, 1987. Elliott's beloved Ann (Phrania Anna Orr Elliott), died in Kerrville on November 11, 1994, at age eighty-nine. According to their wishes, both Fred and Ann Elliott's remains were cremated.

13. Leon Jaworski to Frederick C. Elliott, April 2, 1962; Laurence H. Favrot to Frederick C. Elliott, April 2, 1962; Aris A. Mallas, Jr., to Hines H. Baker, March 19, 1962.

14. Richard E. Wainerdi, interview by William H. Kellar, November 16, 2000; Paul Pendergraft, "Medical Legends," *http://www.kuhf.org,* Houston: KUHF-88.7 FM, 2001.

A NOTE ON SOURCES

The secondary literature used in this study is cited in the notes section that appears at the end of this book. Primary research materials for this history came from several major sources. First, the Texas Medical Center *Annual Report* provided data and follow-up information on many of the people included in Dr. Elliott's manuscript. The John P. McGovern Historical Collections and Research Center in the Houston Academy of Medicine—Texas Medical Center (HAM-TMC) Library is the repository of many audiotapes, videotapes, interview transcripts, and collections of papers and artifacts of Texas Medical Center leaders and founders. Unfortunately, the massive flooding from Tropical Storm Allison in June, 2001, severely damaged the McGovern Archives and much of the collection was destroyed or dislocated. Before the flood, I was fortunate to survey the papers of Drs. Ernst William Bertner, R. Lee Clark, Frederick C. Elliott, Mavis P. Kelsey, Sr., William D. Seybold, and Col. William B. Bates. Along with the papers, oral history interview tapes and transcripts were a key source of information. All collections referred to in the endnotes are found in the McGovern Historical Collections and Research Center unless otherwise noted.

There are three sources of oral history interview tapes and/or transcripts for this project. First, the interviews conducted during 2000–2003 by the author, Dr. William H. Kellar, specifically for this project, which now have been added to the McGovern Historical Collections and Research Center. In addition, during 1973, N. Don Macon conducted a series of videotaped interviews with some of the founders of the Texas Medical Center. And in 1970–71, Dr. William D. Seybold conducted interviews as part of an attempt to establish a Medical Center oral history archive. Interviews with the following people were utilized directly or to provide background information for this project.

INTERVIEWS CONDUCTED BY WILLIAM H. KELLAR

Name	*Date of Interview*
Thomas D. Anderson	January 26, 2000
Paul Gervais Bell	February 27, 2001
J. Searcy Bracewell, Jr.	October 4, 2000

Dr. Chester R. Burns	July 16, 2001
Dr. Denton A. Cooley	December 26, 2000
Dr. Michael E. DeBakey	January 25, 2001
Dr. Mavis P. Kelsey, Sr.	September 19, 2000
	February 7, 2001
Dr. John P. McGovern	February 14, 2000
	April 11, 2000
	May 23, 2000
Dr. Charles H. Oestreich	February 24, 2003
Dr. Ralph Sagebiel	August 7, 2002
Dr. William D. Seybold	November 14, 2000
Dr. William G. Squires, Jr.	July 25, 2002
Dr. Richard E. Wainerdi	November 16, 2000

INTERVIEWS CONDUCTED BY N. DON MACON

Col. William B. Bates	April 19, 1973
Dr. R. Lee Clark	November 30, 1973
Dr. Frederick C. Elliott	July 19, 1973
John H. Freeman	August 2, 1973
Julia Bertner Naylor	July 19, 1973

INTERVIEWS CONDUCTED BY DR. WILLIAM D. SEYBOLD

Dr. Frederick C. Elliott	August 9, 1971
John H. Freeman	April 8, 1971
Anna Hanselman	May 16, 1970

INDEX

Page numbers in *italic* type refer to illustrations.

ABC TV, 156

Abercrombie, J. S., 121–22, 127, 129, 139

Abercrombie, R. H., 127

Academy of Medicine Library, Houston, 91, 94, 129, 134, 147, 158, 170, 182

accreditation, and university affiliation for dental schools, 5, 8

ADA (American Dental Association), 43, 57–58, 60

Airlift, Inc., 166

Allen, Charles, 162

Allen, Charles Channing "Uncle Charley," 30, 31, 32–33

Allen, Raymond B., 89, 91

Alumni Building Company, Texas Dental College, 42, 43

AMA (American Medical Association), 176

Amarillo medical center, 164

American Cancer Society, 155

American Dental Association (ADA), 43, 57–58, 60

American Industrial Hygiene Association, 164

American Medical Association (AMA), 176

American Red Cross, 6, 52–53

Anderson, Clayton & Company, 7, 68, 117, 166, 185

Anderson, James E., 18, 86, 97, 104, 134, 161, 165–66

Anderson, Monroe D. "M. D.": bequests, 180–81, 183; death and foundation establishment, 3, 7, 11, 15, 68, 183; portraits of, 106, 145. *See also* Anderson Foundation

Anderson, T. A., 45

Anderson, Thomas D., 11, 166

Anderson, W. Leland, 18, *90*, 102, 165, 188–94

Anderson Foundation: Baylor Medical College move to Houston, 79, 80–81, 82–83; Bertner Memorial Wing, 135; city-county hospital, 117; Cullen Building, 106; establishment, 3, 7, 8, 81–82, 183–84; Freeman as trustee, 7, 8, 12, 68, 81, 131, 184, 201; Hermann Hospital parking garage, 192; Houston Academy of Medicine library, 94; Joint Administrative Committee, 171; land, 76, 82; Methodist Hospital, 120; St. Joseph Hospital, 180–81; trustees, 7, 8, 11–12, 68, 81, 93, 131, 184, 201; and UT Cancer Foundation, 156; UT Dental Branch building, 72, 79, 109, 131; UT Medical School, Houston, 136–37

Andrews, Jesse L., 111

Arabia (Shrine) Crippled Children's
Hospital, 91, 125, 130, 162
architectural issues: city-county hospi-
tal, 132–33; common building, 169;
Georgia pink marble, TMC, 108,
145; Kipp and TMC, 82, 91, 113–14;
Memorial Center for Health Educa-
tion, vision of, 61–64, *62, 64;* outpa-
tient clinic, 110; TMC plans, 93,
108; UT Dental Branch, 121
Arlington, Kansas, Elliott's work in,
26
Army Corps of Engineers, 105
Arnim, S. S., 125
Arnold, Isaac, 185
Arnold, Joseph, 49
Arnold, Mrs. Isaac, 102
Associates of New Haven, Connecti-
cut, 96–97
Association of American Medical Col-
leges, Council on Medical Educa-
tion, 13, 67
Atlee, R. T., 42
Atomic Energy Commission of
Canada, 165
Audie Murphy Veterans Hospital, San
Antonio, 160
Austin, Texas: single campus proposal
(1943), 84–85; as university site
(1881), 38. *See also* Texas state legis-
lature, Austin; University of Texas
(UT)
Austin American-Statesman, 75, 127
automobile traffic, 113–14, 120, 158,
167, 177–78, 187–88, 200
Aynesworth, Kenneth, 8, 9, 10, 11

Baker, Hines H.: Austin single campus, 85; on Elliott, 208; Elliott for
TMC executive director, 133; TMC
charter, 18, 86; TMC governance
(1940s to 1960s), 98–99, 160, 192; as

UT chancellor candidate, 118; UT
development board, 92
Baker, Rex, 85, 168
Baker Medical Pavilion, Massachu-
setts General Hospital, Boston,
103–104
Ballinger, William Pitt, 9
Baltimore College of Dental Surgery,
Maryland (1840), 38
Baltimore Medical College, Maryland, 38
Bangs, J. L., 128
Bangs, Tina, 128
Baptist Hospital, 181
Barnett, Sue, 97, 135
Bates, William B. "Bill": as Anderson
Foundation trustee, 7, 8, 12, 68;
Buxton Report, 187; on cancer hospital founding, 16; Clark and TMC
board meetings, 99; Elliott's friendship with, 207; Methodist Hospital
expansion, 190–91; Nursing School,
167; Postgraduate Medical Assembly of South Texas, 151; proposed UT cancer hospital in Houston, 68–69; Texas state legislature
funding, 117; and TMC, 18, 86, 87,
88, 192; TMC Medallion awarded
to, 4, *195;* University of Houston
affiliation for Texas Dental College,
6; UT Dental Branch, 47, 71–72,
117
Baylor College of Dentistry, Dallas,
79
Baylor University, Waco, Texas, 17,
80, 171, 173
Baylor University College of Medicine: Clark as dean of, 107–108;
Cullen Building, 87, *101,* 106;
Cullen Foundation, 102, 141; De-
Bakey and Cooley at, 107; Elliott's
imaginary walk through (1976),

200; expansion, 177; Ford Foundation gift, 157; heart research center, 186; Joint Administrative Committee, 171; Mading Foundation, 154; Olson as dean of, 136, 139, 147, 171, 173, 186; outpatient clinic and Bertner, 110; relocation to Houston, 17, 79, 80–81, 82–83; as TMC first medical school, 13–14, 90. *See also* city-county hospital debate; Methodist Hospital, Houston

Bear, Harry, 34

Beard, Norman, 53

beds, TMC hospital, 97, 98, 201

Bellows, Warren, Sr., 93

Ben Taub Hospital, 188, 199

Berconsky, Isaac, 146

Bertelson, Elmer, 136

Bertner, Ernst William "Bill": appointee to Houston Health Department, 55; cancer hospital leadership, 75–78, 83; and Clark, 95, 99; on coordinated medical center, 80, 81; death, 121, 148; Elliott's friendship with, 6–7, 16–17, 207; on flood control, 105; on heating/cooling plant, 102; on Houston state funding projects committee, 116; Institute for Rehabilitation and Research, 200; on institutional cooperation, 103; and Leake, 79–80; M. D. Anderson Cancer Center director, 75–76, 78–79; on Memorial Center for Health Education, 63; Methodist Hospital dedication, 120; Nursing School, 167; outpatient clinic building, 109–10; public health advocacy, 6–7; replacement for, 133; at Rice Hotel, 89; succeeded by Leland Anderson, 166; Texas state legislature lobbying for Dental Branch and TMC (1949–

50), 110–13, 115–19; TMC allocated office space, 145; TMC charter, 18, 86; TMC development, 87–88; as TMC director, 18; TMC institutional plan, 91; as TMC officer, 86; TMC original land parcel deed, *90;* TMC publicity and Barnett, 97; TMC recommendations, Hamilton's, 98; TMC tunnel idea, 172; on UT Dental Branch establishment, 16–17; UT development board, 92–93; UT Public Health School funding, 104–105; vision of medical-educational complex, 3, 156; visiting other medical centers, 103–104; WWII duties, 85; YMCA land request, 106

Bertner, Julia, 134, 148

Bertner Award for Cancer Research, 125–26

Bertner Memorial Wing, M. D. Anderson Cancer Center, 135

Betatron (super x-ray) unit, 132

Bethel, George, 66

Bexar County Medical Society, 159

Birath, Elna: Elliott as TMC executive director, 133–34; Elliott on, 49–51; first meeting with Elliott, 35; Memorial Center for Health Education model placecard holders, 63; on merging dental school with university, 52, 57; Rotary Anns orthodontia clinic, 64; Texas Dental College board reports, 65; on Texas Dental College debt, 51–52; UT Dental Branch, 70, 84–85, 131

Black, Hulon, 91, 92, 93, 194

Blanton, Mr., 70

Blattner, Russell H., 127

Bloom, Fred, 182

Blue Cross/Blue Shield dental operation plan, 57–58

Boardman, Myron, 148

Bonner, Russell, 111

Book of Health, The (Clark, Cumley and Klautz), 141

Boston, Massachusetts General Hospital, 103–104

Bowen, Ted, 138

Bracewell, Searcy, 118–19, 131

Bracket, Anna, 5, 27–28, 29–31

Bradley, Frank R., 147

Branscomb, B. Harvie, 106

Breene, Dr. and Mrs. P. T., 47

Brown, George and Herman, 105

Brown, Herman, 122

Brown, John (Houston physician), 55

Bryan, Dawson, 182

Bryan, Mr. (Second National Bank), 70

budgeting. *See* private funding and philanthropy; Texas state legislature, Austin

buildings. *See specific buildings and institutions*

Bullington, Orville, 85

Bush, Barbara, 208

Butler, P. P., 111

Buxton, Fred, 187

"Buxton Report" on traffic issues, 187

Byrd, Julian, 206

Cady, Lee, 127

Calhoun, John, 8

Calicutt, Laurie, 143

Calvert, Robert S., 112

Calvin, D. Bailey, 73, 74

Canada, Atomic Energy Commission of, 165

Cancer Bulletin, 114–15

cancer center. *See* M. D. Anderson Cancer Center

Cancer Foundation (University of Texas), 93, 119, 156, 200

Carleton, Don E., 9

Carmack, George, 116

cars and traffic, 113–14, 120, 158, 167, 177–78, 187–88, 200

Carter, W. S., 8, 9, 66

Casberg, Melvin A., 167

Casey, Bob, 118, 148

Cato, Arthur, 14–15, 67–68, 69, 70, 121, 148

Cato, Dorothy, 142

Cesium-17 unit, 172–73

Chamber of Commerce, Houston, 6, 46–47, 53, 54, 83, 93–95, 137

Channel 13, Houston ABC affiliate, 156

Chapin, Dr. (historical figure, 1838), 38

charter, TMC, 18–19, 82, 86, 106, 206

Chicago Medical Center, Illinois, 89

Children's Hospital, Shrine Crippled Children's, 91, 125, 130, 162. *See also* Texas Children's Hospital

China, Peking Union Medical College, 10, 67

Chirugien Dentiste oi Traiti des Dents, Le (Fauchard), 38

Christmas Seals, 53

Ciba Corporation, 156

city-county hospital debate: architectural plans (1952), 132–33; Ben Taub Hospital (1961), 188; challenge to (1953), 139, 150–51; Cullen proposals (1949,1956), 114, 153; funding and responsibility arguments (1957–60), 161–62, 163, 176–77, 180; Garrett study (1956), 154–55

City Health Department, 53

Clark, Edward, 163

Clark, J. F., 45

Clark, Jo Lunn, 150–51

Clark, R. Lee: administrative duties, 99; Bertner Award to Stuart, 125–

26; *Book of Health, The* (Clark, Cumley and Klautz), 141; *Cancer Bulletin*, 115; cancer center construction and completion, 122–23, 138, 145; as cancer center director, 95–96, 98–99; Cancer Foundation, 119; Cobalt-60 Irradiator funding, 128; as dean of Baylor School of Medicine, 107–108; Elliott, as post-retirement consultant, 205; and James Anderson, 165; maxillofacial prosthetic department, 120; Texas state legislature lobbying (1940s and 1950s), 99–100, 110–13, 115–19, 137–38; TMC Medallion awarded by, *195;* TMC pink marble building, 108, 145; TMC research expansion, 176

Clayton, Mrs. W. L., 185

Clayton, Will, 7, 187, 191

Cline, Mrs., 70

Cloud, Harry, 46, 47

cobalt-60 irradiator, 128, 130, 132, 165

Cobb, Beatrix, 142, 143

Cobb, William, 144–45

Cody, Claude C., Jr., 134, 146, 178

Cody, Mrs. Claude, 134

College of Dental Nursing, 90

Collins, Al, 109

Committee of 75 (Texas Exes), 168–69

Committee of 100 (Texas Exes), 92–93, 100

commons building idea, 169–70, 191

communication within TMC, 110

Community Chest, Houston, 52, 53, 54

Coogle, C. P., 76

Cooley, Denton A., 19, 107, 150

Cooley, Ralph C., 18, 19, 45

cooling/heating plant, TMC utilities, 93, 102, 193

Copeland, Murray, 183

Council on Dental Education, American Dental Association, 43, 60

Council on Medical Education, Association of American Medical Colleges, 13, 67

county issues. *See* Harris County, Texas

Coyle, Tom, 48

Crone, E. M., 48

Cronkite, Walter, Jr., 49

Cronkite, Walter, Sr., 48–49

Crossland, Kathryn, 183

Crump, Houston, 111

Culberson, Charles Allen, 38

Cullen, (Hugh) Roy: on city-county hospital, 114, 150, 153; Cullen Building, 106; foundation established, 101–102; Hugh Roy Cullen Day, 148; Jefferson Davis Hospital into tuberculosis hospital, 114; outpatient clinic funding, 106, 109–10; portrait, 106; St. Luke's Hospital, 141, 147–48, 185; as TMC trustee, 89

Cullen, Lillie, 102, 106, 141, 147–48

Cullen Building, *10,* 87, 106

Cullen Foundation gifts, 101–102, 106, 109–10, 114, 117, 120, 141

Cullinan, Craig, 116

Cullinan, J. S., II, 166

Cullinan, Nina, 166

Cumley, Russell, 114–15, 141

Cutrer, Louis, 166, 177

Daily, Ray K., 6

Dallas medical school proposal (1949), 112

Daniel, Price, 148

Daniels, Bill, 136, 138

David Runyon Memorial Fund, 128

Davis, Gene, 153

DeBakey, Michael, 107, 176, 183

Dental Nursing, College of, 90

dental schools: accreditation and university affiliation, 5, 8; Baltimore College of Dental Surgery (1840), 38; Baylor College of Dentistry, Dallas, 79; Galveston medical school consideration (1895), 38; Kansas City Dental College, 5, 29, 31, 32, 50, 51. *See also* Texas Dental College; University of Texas Dental Branch

"Dentist of the Century" award to Elliott, 174–75

Department of Health, Education and Welfare (HEW), 171, 172

Department of Preventive Medicine, Baylor University College of Medicine, 189–90

Depression, 50–51, 53

Dickson, Charles, 166

Disney, Walt, 31, 129

Distinguished Service Medal, AMA, for DeBakey, 176

Division of Cancer Research, state funding (1941), 15

Dixon, J. Charles, 115

Dmochowski, Leon, 155

doctors. *See specific persons; specific topics*

Doctor's Club, TMC, 145–46

"Doctor's Office, The" (KXYZ radio), 53

drugstore work, Elliott's, 4–5, 22, 24–29

Dudley, Ray L., 18, 86, 106, 128

Durham, Mylie, Sr., 55

Duval, Representative, 43–44

Eastwood, Richard T., 189, 190, 191–94

Edge, Charles, 48

education. *See specific topics*

Edwards, Ralph, 151

Eisenhower, Dwight D., 146

Elkins, James A., Jr., 122

Elkins, Wilson H., 95

Ellerbe Company, 188

Elliott, Anna Bracket (first wife), 5, 27–28, 29–31

Elliott, Annie (aunt), 21

Elliott, Ann Orr (second wife): on Cullens, 141; loss of Scherer and Hight, 127; Memphis lab assistance, 33; retirement years, 194–95, 204–205, *205;* as TMC executive director's wife, 134, *140;* on WWII, 70–71, 86–87

Elliott, Chesley (sister), 22

Elliott, Francis "Frank" (brother), 22, 24–26, *25,* 28

Elliott, Frederick Chesley "Fred," 174–75; adolescence and young adulthood, 25–28; as Anderson Foundation trustee, 201; Bertner friendship, 6–7, 207; on Birath, 49–51; birth and childhood (1865), 4–5; cancer center ground breaking, 122–23; cancer hospital first clinical staff (1943), 78; childhood, 21–26, *23;* commons building idea, 169–70; death, 19, 205; dental training, 5, 29–30, 32; as "Dentist of the Century," 174–75; drugstore and pharmacy work, 4–5, 22, 24–29; on early TMC cooperation and coordination, 98, 103, 160–61; eulogized as a visionary, 205–208; Fouchard Gold Medal, 187; as founder, TMC, 4, 7–8; honors, Texas Lutheran College, 202–204; illness, 140–41; imaginary walk through Texas Medical Center (1976), 199; as lecturer, UTMB, 10–11, 67, 73–74; life summary, 174–75; marriage to, and death of, Anna Bracket, 5, 27–28,

39–31; marriage to Anna Orr, 32; as Max Krost Charitable Trust trustee, 201, 203; member, Texas State Board of Health, 59, 74–75; on mother's letter regarding TMC, 197–99; professor, University of Tennessee College of Dentistry, 5, 32–34, 97; and Rainey, *94;* retirement, 188–89, 193–96, 200, 201, 204–205, 206, 207–208; on San Antonio medical center, 158–60; as Texas Dental College dean, 3, 5–6, 8, 34–36, *36,* 48–83, *65;* Texas state legislature lobbying (1940s and 1950s), 16–17, 66–67, 69–70, 76–78, 111–19; TMC establishment and charter, 18–19, 86; as TMC executive director, 133–35, *140,* 145–46, *169,* 207; TMC governance plan, 160–61; TMC Medallion awarded to, 4, *195;* as TMC trustee, 86, 200; as UT Dental Branch dean, 3, 16, 83–84, 95, 130–31, 134; as vice president, UT, 94–95; vision for public health, 3–4, 202, 203; vision for TMC, 4, 7–8, 169–70, 173–74. *See also* University of Texas Dental Branch

Elliott, James (grandfather), 21, 22
Elliott, Ray (no relationship), 165
Elliott, Ruth (aunt), 21
Elliott, Sarah (grandmother), 21
Elliott, Thomas Amos (father), 21, 22–27, *25*
Elsevier Press, 141
e-ray (Betatron) unit, 132
Ewalt, Jack, 121, 142
Exxon, 92
eye institute in TMC, 113, 178
Eyes of Texas Foundation, 164–65

Farfel, Bernard, 185
Fauchard, Pierre, 4, 38

Fauchard Academy, 4
Favrot, Laurence H., 192, 207–208
Favrot Building, 199
financial issues. *See* private funding and philanthropy; Texas state legislature, Austin
First Methodist Church, 182
First National Bank, 59, 95, 111
First United Methodist Church, 162
First World War, 29–30
Fitzgerald, Winnie, 49
Fleming, Lamar, 7, 122
Fleming, Lamar, Jr., 162
Fletcher, Gilbert, 128, 130, 132, 165
flooding, TMC, 105
flu (influenza) pandemic, 30–31
Fondren, Mrs. Walter W., 115, 185
Fonville, R. H., 54–55
Ford Foundation, 157
Foster, Joe B., 78
Foster, John H., 78
Fouchard Gold Medal, 187
foundations. *See* private funding and philanthropy
Fox, Thomas P., 187
Franco, Francisco, 146
Frankl, Viktor E., 181
Fransworth and Chamber's Construction Company, 127
Franzheim, R. Kenneth, 172, 173
Frederick C. Elliott Chair in Health Fitness and Nutrition, Texas Lutheran College, Seguin, 204
Freeman, John H.: as Anderson Foundation trustee, 7, 8, 12, 68, 81, 131, 184, 201; on Austin single campus, 84–85; Elliott's friendship with, 201, 207; Joint Administrative Committee, 171; as Max Krost Charitable Trust trustee, 201, 203; M.D. Anderson Hospital, 15–16, 148; Postgraduate Medical Assembly of

Freeman, John H. (*cont.*)
South Texas lunch, 151; Rice Hotel, 89; Shrine Crippled Children's Hospital, 125, 130; TMC charter, 18, 86; TMC naming, 81; TMC publicity, 86; as TMC trustee, 86; UT Dental Branch, 16, 131; visiting other medical centers, 103–104

Freud, Sigmund, 181

Fuerman, George, 114–15, 119

Fulbright, Crooker, Freeman & Bates, 7

funding. *See* private funding and philanthropy; public funding

"Future Development of the University of Texas, The" (Rainey), 84–85

Galveston, Texas: dental school proposal (1927–31), 44–48; medical school (1956–90), 37, 38. *See also* University of Texas Medical Branch (UTMB), Galveston

Galveston News, 44

Gambati, Olympio F., 40, 42

Gamm, Lee II, 139

Garrett, Ross, 154–55

Garrison, Monte, 54

Garrott, Helen Holt, 157–58

Geographic Medicine, Institute of, 80, 90, 109, 110

Georgetown University, Washington, D.C., 34

Georgia pink marble, TMC, 108, 145

Gerontology, Institute of, 80, 90

Girard, Louis, 165

Girls' Home School, 53–54

Gladstone, William Ewart, 21

Glasco, Kansas, Elliott's work in, 28–29

Goar, E. L., 78

Goldson, Mrs. Walter, 115

Good Samaritan Club and building, 162, 169–70, 174

Gottlieb, Dr. (TMC pathology faculty), 181

Gray, M. L., 115

Great Depression, 50–51, 53

Green, Charles, 115

Greensburg, Kansas, Elliott's work in, 27

Greenville *Morning Herald,* 112

Greenwood, James A., 78, 174

Greer, David, 78, 99, 139

Gregory, Raymond, 80

Gresham, Newton, 191

Griffey, Edward, 113

Griffin, A. Clark, 186

Griffing, Burrell, 33

Grimmett, Dr. (TMC nuclear medicine faculty), 128, 165

Griswold, C. M., 78

Guillemin, Roger, 153–54, 183

Guinn, John, 168, 193

Gulf Coast Medical Foundation, 156

Gulf Sulphur Company, 111

Gurley, Helen and Webb, 34

H. D. Justi Tooth Manufacturing Company, 32

Halmark, Mollie, 193

Hamilton, James A., 96, 97–98, 104

Hamm, Goldie, 55

Hamrick, Wendell, 180

Hankamer, Earl C., 128, 171

Hanselman, Anna, 78, 185

Hardin, Carl, 69, 74, 76–78, 118

Harding College, Arkansas, 184

Harris, Dr. (historical figure, 1838), 38

Harris, Herbert, 166

Harris, Titus, 75

Harris County, Texas: Charity Hospital, 188; Medical Society, 40, 94, 111, 137, 149, 180; Morgue, 163. *See also* city-county hospital debate

Hart, James P., 118, 126, 130, 131, 133–34, 137, 138

Haviland, Kansas, Elliott's work in, 27–28, *28*

Hayes, Herbert T., 78

Health League of Texas, 59

heating/cooling plant, TMC utilities, 93, 102, 193

Heflebower, Roy C., 185

Heitman, F. A., 47

heliport, 166

Hermann Hospital: adjacent to TMC, 87; Bertner at, 78; Cullen Foundation gifts, 102; Junior League of Houston, 128–29; new building for, 96, 110–11; parking, 192; and TMC, 13, 14, 16, 17–18, 90; U of H School of Practical Nursing, 120

Hermann Park, 17–18

Hermann Professional Building, 96, 145

Hermann University (1844), 37

HEW (Department of Health, Education and Welfare), 171, 172

Hight, Finis M., 35, 36, 43–44, 47, 48, 65–66, 127

Hill, George A., Jr., 89–91, 92, 100, 110

Hilltop Village Nursing Home, Kerrville, Texas, 205

Hinds, E. C., 126

HISD (Houston Independent School District), 6, 54

Hite, Rosalie B., 100

Hobby, Oveta Culp, 89, 113, 172

Hobby, William Pettus, 116

Hofheinz, Ray, 145, 148

Hogg, James S., 17

Hogg, Will C., 17, 81

Hogg Foundation, 143

Holcombe, Oscar, 105, 106, 114, 130–31

Hollers, James "Jim," 159–60

Holt, Helen, 157–58

Hoover Commission Report, 113

House Bill 190 (1897), Texas, 39

House Bill 268 (1941), Texas, 14

House Bill 279 (1943), Texas, 76–77, 78

Houston, Horace, Jr., 136

Houston, Texas: Baylor University College of Medicine relocation to, 17, 79, 80–81, 82–83; Board of Health, 6, 63; Chamber of Commerce, 6, 46–47, 53, 54, 83, 93–95, 137; City Council, 54–57; Community Chest, 52, 53, 54; Elliott's arrival, 48–49; Elliott's public health advocacy, 3–4, 6; as fastest growing city in U.S. (1952), 132; population (1930s), 5; Public Health Department, 6, 54–59, 189; rejected as state medical school site (1881), 38; State Psychiatric Hospital, 187; TMC economic impact on, 155, 200; University of Houston, 6, 90, 102, 105, 120, 136, 167, 184; University of St. Thomas, 184. *See also* city-county hospital debate; *specific topics*

Houston Academy of Medicine Library, 91, 94, 129, 134, 147, 158, 170, 182

Houston Anti-Tuberculosis League, 53

Houston Business, 155

Houston Chronicle: on city-county hospital debate, 150–51; on Elliott's arrival, 48; on Elliott's life, 174–75; on Elliott's vision, 169–70, 173–74; on Texas state legislature TMC funding, 109, 111–12, 115–16; on Texas Women's University School of Nursing, 168; on TMC accomplishments (1954), 145; on TMC tunnel, 172; on traffic in TMC, 166–67

Houston Council of Social Agencies, 52, 53, 54

Houston District Dental Society, 4, 57–58

Houston Endowment, 171, 182

Houston Independent School District (HISD), 6, 54

Houston Magazine, 46–47

Houston Negro Hospital, 166

Houston Oil Company, 92

Houston Pediatric Society, 99

"Houston Plan" for dental care, 58–59

Houston Post, 48, 83, 87, 94, 116, 149, 150–51, 168, 177

Houston Rotary Club, 4, 54

Houston Safety Association, American Red Cross, 52–53

Howard, Philo, 55

Hughes, Howard, 101, 142, 163

Hugh Roy Cullen: A Story of American Opportunity (Kilman and Wright), 148

Humble Oil and Refining Company, 92, 118, 129, 161

Hurley, Marvin, 131

Hurricane Carla (1962), 191

Hurricane of 1900, Galveston, 17

Hyman, Dr. (University of Tennessee VP), 164

India, Tata Memorial Hospital, Bombay, 10, 15, 67

Industrial Hygiene Association, 164

infantile paralysis (polio), 6, 53, 136, 179

influenza pandemic, 30–31

Institute for Rehabilitation and Research, 162, 200

Institute of Geographic Medicine, 80, 90, 109, 110

Institute of Gerontology, 80, 90

Institute of Orthodontics, 90

Institute of Rehabilitative Medicine, NYU Medical Center, 80

Institute of Religion, 154, 177, 181–82, 200

insurance, Blue Cross/Blue Shield dental operation plan, 57–58

Irving, George M., 171

Jachimczyk, Joseph A., 163

Jackson, J. M., 97, 131–32

James A. Hamilton and Associates, Connecticut, 96

Jaworski, Leon, 170–71, 207

Jeffers, Leroy, 167–68

Jefferson Davis Hospital, 53, 104, 114, 120, 155, 162, 164

Jenness, Isaac (uncle), 21

Jenness, Katherine (mother), 21–24

Jenness, Mr. (grandfather), 22

Jesse H. Jones building, 171

Jesse H. Jones library, 91, 94, 129, 134, 147, 158, 170, 182

Jesse H. Jones Physical Education Complex, Texas Lutheran College, Seguin, 202

Jewish Community of Houston, 171

Jewish Medical Research Institute and building, 171, 177, 178, 185

John Freeman Building, 199

John Sealy Hospital, Galveston, 9, 11, 12

Johnson, Bob, 111

Johnson, Jack, 131

Johnson, Marshall G. and Lilli, 156, 184, 199–201, 202, 204

Johnson and Maddox, 110

Johnson Foundation, 199–200, 201, 202, 204

Johnson Health and Fitness Center, Texas Lutheran College, Seguin, 202

Johnston, Robert A., 78

Joint Administrative Committee, 171

Jones, Bush, 45

Jones, Jesse H., 6, 89, 94, 116, 127, 147, 182

Jones, John, 168, 171, 193

Jones, Margaret, 83

Jones, Mrs. Jesse, 134

Junior League of Houston, 128–29, 184

Kahn, Eugene, 143

Kamrath, Karl, 108

Kansas City, Kansas, Elliott's work in, 5, 29–32, 50–51

Kansas City Dental College, 5, 29, 31, 32, 50, 51

Kelsey, Mavis P., Sr., 19, 132, 136–37

Kelsey-Seybold Clinic, 19

Kerr, Denton, 111

Kerrville, Texas, Elliott's retirement to, 204–206

Kessler, George, 162

Kilman, Ed, 148

Kimbro, Robert W., 180

Kipp, H. A., 82, 91, 113–14

Kirby, John Henry, 40, 47

Kirkland, William A., 59–60, 95, 171, 192

Kirschbaum, Arthur, 146–47, 165

Kiwanis Club, 87

Klautz, John P., 141

Klein, Mr. and Mrs. Nathan, 135

Knutson Construction Company, 162

Krost, Max, 201. *See also* Max Krost Charitable Trust

Krost Life Enrichment Program, Texas Lutheran College, Seguin, 203

KXYZ radio, Houston, 53

land: San Antonio medical center, 158–60; 1940's issues, 13, 14, 16, 17–18, *90*, 91, 104–6; 1950's issues, 158, 167–68; 1969's issues, 191, 193

Law, Francis M., 201

Leach, Sayles, 171

Leake, Chauncey D.: cancer hospital development, 76; Clark meeting, 95; on commons building idea, 170; *Houston Post* story on early Texas medicine (1955), 149–50; Institute of Geographic Medicine, 110; Jesse H. Jones building, 147; Texas Dental College budget, 86; TMC plans, 82, 91; UT development board, 92–93; UTMB, 13, 76, 79–80, 95

Leake, J. W., Jr., 122

Le Chirugien Dentiste oi Traiti des Dents (Fauchard), 38

Ledbetter, Paul V., 146, 151

legislature, state. *See* Texas state legislature, Austin

Levinson, Rosalie, 193–94

Levy, M. D., 78

Levy, Moise, 94, 134, 146

Lhamon, William, 143, 176, 181, 187

library, Houston Academy of Medicine, 91, 94, 129, 134, 147, 158, 170, 182

Lions Club, 165

Loock, Mr. (maintenance man), 131

Lubbock medical school, Texas, 164

Lutheran Hospital Association, 173

Lutheran Hospital Center, 173, 184

Lutheran Pavilion Building, 184, 199–200, 201

M. D. Anderson Building, 171

M. D. Anderson Cancer Center: Anderson Foundation support for, 13, 14, 16, 17, 68–69; Bertner as director, 75–76, 78–79; building construction (1940s and 1950s), 93, 121, *122*, 122–23, 128, 138, 145; Cesium-17 unit, 172–73; cobalt-60 irradiator, 128, 130, 132, 165; Elliott as post-

M. D. Anderson Cancer Center (*cont.*)
retirement consultant to, 200, 204,
205; Elliott's imaginary walk past
(1976), 199–200; expansion, 135,
154, 186; founding, 13, 15–16; Hites
funds, 100; staffing, 83; Texas state
legislature lobbying (1940s and
1950s), 13–17, 67–68, 69, 111–19,
137–38, 141–42; as UT cancer hospi-
tal, 13, 14, 16, 17, 68–69, 90
M. D. Anderson Foundation. *See* An-
derson Foundation
McAshan, Mrs., 187–88, 191
McCaleb, Dr. (University of Ten-
nessee faculty), 33
McCarty, Glen, 127–28
McCarty, W. B., 45
McFarland, Ike, 53
McGee, Vernon, 144
MacKie, Fred, 108
MacKie and Kamrath, 121
McNaughton, Aileen, 35
Macon, N. Don, 5, 205
Mallas, Aris A., Jr., 208
March Culmore Hall, 193, 199
March of Dimes, 53
Marine Hospital, 104, 113
Markwell, Russell, 45
Marshall, Douglas B., 102
Marshall G. and Lillie Johnson Foun-
dation, 199–200, 201, 202, 204
Martha G. Dunn Memorial Chapel,
199
Massachusetts General Hospital,
103–104
Massachusetts General Hospital,
Boston, 103–104
Massey, Otis, 56
maxillofacial prosthetic department,
120
Max Krost Charitable Trust, 201, 202,
203–204

Maxwell House coffee, 94
Mayo Clinic, Minnesota, 104
Mayo Foundation, 176
Medical College of Virginia, Richmond, 34
medical education. *See specific colleges
and universities*
"Medical Horizons" (television, 1956),
156
Melnick, Joseph, 179
Memorial Center for Health Educa-
tion, vision of, 7–8, 17, 61–64, *62,
64*
Memorial Hospital, Houston, 181
Memphis, University of Tennessee
College of Dentistry, 5, 32–34, 50,
51, 97
mental health care: Houston State
Psychiatric Hospital, 187; Texas
Research Institute of Mental Sciences, 144–45, 157–58, 163–64, 177,
200
mental/intellectual life, importance of
care for, 199
Merchant, M. S., 38, 40, 41–42
Methodist Church, Texas Annual
Conference of, 161
Methodist Hospital, Houston: administrators Roberts and Bowen,
138; construction and dedication,
90–91, 96, 102, 115, 120, 129; Cullen
Foundation gifts, 102; Daniels' visit,
136, 138; Elliott's imaginary walk
past (1976), 199; expansion (1950s
and 1960s), 154, 161, 184–85, 191;
land deed restriction issues, 105;
medical photographer Davis, 153;
polio, 53; U of H School of Practical Nursing, 120. *See also* Baylor
University College of Medicine
Methodist Hospital, San Antonio, 159
Methodist Hospital Foundation, 161

Meyer, Leopold L. "Lep," 122, 127, 129, 139, 155
mice for research (1954), 146–47
Midgely, Albert, 47
monorail idea, 158, 167, 177–78
Montgomery Ward gift, 131
Moore, Senator, 77–78
Morrison, Earl, 186–87
Moursund, Walter, 81, 136, 173
Mumford, David M., 206
Murphy, Marcus, 131
Murrow, Wright, 147, 148
Musgrove, John, 78
Muskogee, Oklahoma, Elliott's work in, 26

National Heart Institute, 186
National Institutes of Health, 177, 179
Neal, J. W., 94
Newton Rayzor Building, 171
New York University Medical Center, Institute of Rehabilitative Medicine, 80
Nixon, Patricia "Pat," 155
noise pollution, TMC, 164
Norseman, O. L., 115
Northwest University, 131
nursing: College of Dental, 90; Hamilton on, 98; School of Practical Nursing, University of Houston, 120; Texas Women's University School of, 168, 169, 172, 182–83, 191, 193, 199; TMC school for, 162; UT school for, 167–68

Oates, L. S., 129
O'Daniel, W. Lee, 15, 59
Oestreich, Charles H., 203
Olson, John V., 134, 135, 137, 151, 206
Olson, Stanley, 136, 139, 147, 171, 173, 186
Olson, Victor, 192

ophthalmology, eye institute in TMC, 113, 178
Orr, Phrania Anna "Ann," 5, 32. See also Elliott, Ann Orr (second wife)
orthodontia clinic and Rotary Anns, 64, 132
Orthodontics, Institute of, 90
outpatient clinic, 105–6, 109–10

Painter, Theophilus S., 13, 95, 100, 123, 137–38
Parker, Virginia, 158
parking, 187–88, 190, 192, 200
Parten, J. R., 8, 10, 11, 92
Patton, W. S., 53
Peking Union Medical College, China, 10, 67
Perry, Glenn, 105, 150
Petersen, Henry, 55, 63–64
pharmacy work, Elliott's, 4–5, 22, 24–29
Phelps, Edward S., 40
philanthropy. See private funding and philanthropy
Phillips, J. A., 47
physical life, importance of care for, 199
physicians. See specific persons; specific topics
Pierre Fauchard Academy, 4, 187
pink marble, TMC, 108, 145
Pittsburg, Kansas, 21–26, 27–28, 31
Pittsburgh, Pennsylvania, University Cathedral of Learning, 7–8, 61, 62
Pitzer, Kenneth S., 195
polio, 6, 53, 136, 179
political issues: leadership conflict at UTMB, 8–13, 73–75, 77; UT leadership conflict, 8, 10–13, 77. See also city-county hospital debate; Texas state legislature, Austin
Portanova, Lillie Cranz, 102

portraits: of Anderson, 106, 145; of Cullens, 106; of Elliott, 192
Poster, John H., 78, 115
Poster, Joseph, 53
Postgraduate Medical Assembly of South Texas, 151
Postgraduate Medical School, 90, 162–63, 181, 191
Potter, Hugh, 47
Powers, George, 34–35, 43
Prentice-Hall Publishers, 148
Pressler, Herman P., 122
Preventive Medicine, Department of, Baylor University College of Medicine, 189–90
private funding and philanthropy: American Red Cross, 6, 52–53; Cancer Foundation, UT, 93, 119, 156, 200; Christmas Seals, 53; Committee of 75 (Texas Exes), 168–69; Committee of 100 (Texas Exes), 92–93, 100; David Runyon Memorial Fund, 128; Eyes of Texas Foundation, 164–65; Fuerman gift, 119–20; Good Samaritan Club and building, 162, 169–70, 174; Hite gift, 100; Hughes proposed gift (1954), 142; Jesse H. Jones Foundation, 182; Johnson Foundation, 199–200, 201, 202, 204; Junior League of Houston, 128–29, 184; Klein gift, 135; Knutson gift, 162; Mading Foundation, 154; March of Dimes, 53; Marshall G. and Lillie Johnson Foundation, 199–200, 201, 202, 204; Mayo Foundation, 176; Purchase gift, 93; Rotary Anns, 64, 132; Rotary Club, 86; Texaco gift, 179; Texas Children's Foundation, 122; Texas Exes, 92–93, 100, 168–69; Whittington gift, 117. *See also* Anderson Foundation

Prudential Insurance Company building, 119, 128, 136
Pruitt, Raymond D., 174
psychiatric care, Texas Research Institute of Mental Sciences, 144–45, 157–58, 163–64, 177, 200
public funding, 153, 171, 172, 185, 186. *See also* private funding and philanthropy; Texas state legislature, Austin
public health: Bertner advocacy, 6–7; Elliott's vision for, 3–4, 202, 203; Houston Public Health Department, 54–59, 189; Texas Lutheran College, Seguin, 201–204; Texas State Board of Health, 6, 59, 74–75, 140; UT School of Public Health, 90, 104–105, 110. *See also specific topics*
Pullen, Roscoe, 132
Purchase, Mr. and Mrs. Norman, 93

Quin, Clinton S., 18, 53–54, 86, *90*, 129, 147–48
Quin, Mrs. Clinton, 53–54

Radio Corporation of America, 156
radio KXYZ, 53
Rainey, Homer P.: Austin single campus, 84–85; Bertner for cancer hospital leadership, 75; cancer hospital founding, 15–16; and Elliott, *94;* Leake support, 80; on UT Dental Branch, 70, 74, 77–78; UTMB conflict, 10, 11, 12, 13, 77; UT vs. Baylor affiliation, 79
Randall, Edward, 8–10, 11, 12, 15, 47, 73
Rayzor, Mr. and Mrs. Newton, 171, 183
Rayzor Student Center, 183
real estate. *See* architectural issues; land; *specific buildings*
Red Cross, American, 6, 52–53

Rehabilitation and Research, Institute for, 162, 200
Religion, Institute of, 154, 181–82, 200
religious life, importance of care for, 199
Renis, Emmiline, 53
research mice (1954), 146–47
retirement, Elliott's, 188–89, 193–96, 200, 201, 204–205, *206,* 207–208
Rice Hotel, 18, 89, 162
Rice Institute, 52, 59–60, 61, 90, 95, 105, 136, 184
Rice Institute Cooperative Program for Research, 90
Rice University, 195
Richmond, Fred, 151
Richmond, Medical College of Virginia, 34
Rider, Ed, 116–17
Ripley Foundation, 63
roads and streets, TMC, 113–14, 120, 158, 167, 177–78, 187–88, 200
Roberts, Josie, 96, 115, 138
Robertson, Mrs. Corbin, 102
Robinson, Hampton, 140
Robinson, James, 174
Robinson, Robert "Bob," 35, 62–63
Rockefeller Foundation, 10, 67, 177
Rockwell, James, 131
Rosalie B. Hite bequest (1946), 100
Rotary Anns, 64, 132
Rotary Club, 86
Rowsey, Luther, 148–49
Royall, Kenneth C., 106
Roy G. Cullen Building, UH, 102
Ruilman, Cyril J., 163–64, 176
Runyon Memorial Fund, 128
Rusk, Howard A., 80
Russell, William, 163

Sabin, Albert, 179
St. Joseph's Hospital, 125, 180–81

St. Luke's Hospital: Cullen Foundation, 102; dedication, 141, 147–48, 185; Elliott's imaginary walk past (1976), 199; expansion, 185; fund drive, 100; land deed restriction issues, 105; TMC dedication, 90
St. Paul's Methodist Church, 182
St. Thomas University, Houston, 184
Sakowitz, 164–65
Salk, Jonas, 149
Salk vaccine, 179
San Antonio Medical Foundation, 159
San Antonio medical school proposal, 110, 112, 158–60
Saville, David, 166
Scherer, Walter H., 35, 40, 42, 47, 66–67, 71–72, 74, 127
Schlenk, Fritz, 76
School of Practical Nursing, University of Houston, 120
Sealy, John, 9
Sealy, John II, 9
Sealy, Tom, 129, 138, 148
Sealy and Smith Foundation, 9
Second National Bank, 70
Second World War, 15–18, 71–75, 86–87
Seguin, Texas, Texas Lutheran College, 201–204
Senate Bill 114 (1895), Texas, 39
Senate Bill 217 (1895), Texas, 39
Senterfitt, Rueben, 136
Seventy-five Year History (of UTMB), 11
Shamrock Hotel, 105
Shenkler, Irvin, 177
Shivers, Allan, 115–16, 126–27, 141–44, 148, 187
Shrine Crippled Children's Hospital, 91, 125, 130, 162
Simmons, Carroll D., 83–84, 192

Sinclair, W. K., 165
Slaughter, Don, 73
Smith, Ashbel, 37
Smith, Bob, 162, 170
Smith, E. W., 45, 48
Smith, Frank A., 115
Smith, Jennie Sealy, 9
Smith, Stanley L., 129
Smith, William A., 122
Snider, Raymond, 35
Soule University (closed, 1856), 37
Southern Pacific Hospital, 125
Southern Pacific Railroad, 125
South Texas Medical Center, San Antonio, 159
Southwestern Medical School, UT Dallas, 168
Sparenberg, Charles, 83–84
Speech and Hearing Center, 128, 164, 166
Spies, John W., 8, 10–15, 66–70, 73–76, 80
Spies, Tom D., 10, 66
State National Bank of Houston, 18
State Psychiatric Institute for Mental Sciences, 142–45, 157–58, 163–64, 177, 200
streets and roads, TMC, 113–14, 120, 158, 167, 177–78, 187–88, 200
Strickland, D. F., 85
Stuart, Fred, 125–26
students, TMC growth (1963–2000), 201. See also specific topics
Sutherland, Robert, 143
Sutherland, W. T., 128

Talbot, W. O., 39, 44, 46, 54
Tata Memorial Hospital, Bombay, India, 10, 15, 67
Taylor, Grant, 162, 190–91
Taylor, Judson L., 55, 66, 75–76, 78, 107

TB (tuberculosis) hospital, 53, 91, 107, 114, 150
Tejml, Emil, 65
telethon, eye institute, 165
Television, TMC, 102
"Television Facilities" UT Dental Branch, 186–87
Tellepsen, Howard, 127
Tellepsen Construction Company, 127
Tellepson, Howard, 164
Texaco, 179
Texas A&M College, 80, 184
Texas Annual Conference of the Methodist Church, 161
Texas Children's Foundation, 122
Texas Children's Hospital: Abercrombie fund raising, 121–22; Anderson, Clayton and Company endowment, 185; dedication, 138; Disney brochure for, 129; Elliott's imaginary walk past, 199; groundbreaking, 127; Junior League of Houston, 129; land deed restriction issues, 105; Pat Nixon's visit to, 155
Texas Dental College: board meetings, 64–65; closure, and UT Dental Branch begun (1943), 72, 74, 83–84; Elliott as dean, 3, 5–6, 8, 34–36, 36, 48–83, 65; establishment and early years (1905–32), 43f, 44f, 45f, 46f, 49–48; financial challenges, 48–51; orthodontia clinic, 64; university affiliation sought, 5–6, 8, 46–47, 51–52; UT Dental Branch established, 13, 16, 66, 67
Texas Dental Society, 45–46, 48
Texas Exes (UT alumni), 92–93, 100, 168–69
Texas Heart Institute, 199
Texas Lutheran College (now University), Seguin, Texas, 201–204
Texas Medical Association, 14, 15, 180

"Texas Medical Center News," 148–49
Texas Medical Center News, The (1946–53), 97
Texas Medical Center Research Society, 181
Texas Medical Center (TMC): 1941–1946, 13–18; 1946–1948, 89–108; 1948–1950, 109–24; 1951–1955, 125–52; 1956–1959, 153–78; 1960–1963, 179–98; aerial photograph (2002), *197;* Baylor Medical College, 79, 80–81, 82–83; brochure on UT programs in TMC, 92–93; charter, 18–19, 82, 86, 106, 206; city-county hospital, 114–15; commons building idea, 169–70, 191; cooperation and coordination, 98, 103, 160–61; Cullen Foundation, 102; dedication, 18, 89, *90;* Elliott as trustee, 86, 200; Elliott honored, 4; Elliott's imaginary walk past (1976), 199; Elliott's proposal to have Houston public health department in, 189–90; Elliott's retirement, 188, 193–94, 200, 201, 204; Elliott's vision, 169–70, 173–74; flood control, 105; governance plan, 160–61, 189; growth (2000), 200; Joint Administrative Committee, 171; land for UT cancer hospital in Houston, 14; "Medical Center Visitation Day" (May 9,1954), 145; mother's letter regarding, 197–99; naming, 81; nursing school, 162; planning for, 91, 208; research expansion, 176, 186–87; research recognition, 179, 183; trustee actions, early, 94–99, 104–7; UT Medical School, Houston, 90, 132, 136–37, 199; vision of, 207–8; worth to Houston, 87–88. *See also* Baylor University College of Medicine

Texas Research Institute of Mental Sciences, 142–45, 157–58, 163–64, 177, 200
Texas State Board of Dental Examiners, 38, 40, 69
Texas State Board of Dental Society, 48
Texas State Board of Health, 6, 59, 74–75, 140
Texas State Cancer Hospital, 15. *See also* M. D. Anderson Cancer Center
Texas State Dental Association, 54
Texas State Dental Society, 69
Texas State Department of Health, 14
Texas State Hospital Board, 54, 187
Texas state legislature, Austin: dental practice regulation (1895, 1897, 1919), 39; dental school as university affiliate (1931), 39–40, 46–48; dental school funding (1895,1927), 39, 43–44; Elliott and Clark to (1946), 99–100; House Bill 190 (1897), 39; House Bill 268 (1941), 14; House Bill 279 (1943), 76–77, 78; Houston visit by, 100, 136; M. D. Anderson Cancer Center funding (1940s and 1950s), 13–17, 67–68, 69, 111–19, 137–38, 141–42; Senate Bill 114 (1895), 39; Senate Bill 217 (1895), 39; Texas Research Institute of Mental Sciences, 144–45, 157; TMC funding (1949,1950,1953), 111–13, 115–17, 118–19, 136–37, 141–42; university and medical school approval (1881), 37–38; UT cancer hospital legislation, 13, 14–16, 17, 67–70, 69; UT Dental Branch (1941–43), 16–17, 66–67, 69–70, 76–78; UT Dental Branch (1940s and 1950s), 13, 16–17, 66–67, 69–71, 76–78, 111–13, 115–19, 126–27; UT institutions and operations at TMC, 100, 137–40; UTMB improvements, 14–15, 66–70, 73

Texas State Psychiatric Hospital, 187

Texas Women's University School of Nursing in Texas Medical Center, 168, 169, 172, 182–83, 191, 193, 199

Thomas, Albert, 113

Thomas F. Ellerbe Company, 110

TMC. *See* Texas Medical Center (TMC)

traffic issues, 113–14, 120, 158, 167, 177–78, 187–88, 200

Transient Relief Committee, 53

Truman, Harry, 93

tuberculosis (TB) hospital, 53, 91, 107, 114, 150

tunnel plan, 171–72, 188

Turner, Ben Weems, 78

unit method of study, 82

University of Houston, Texas, 6, 90, 102, 105, 120, 136, 167, 184

University of Minnesota, 104

University of Pittsburgh Cathedral of Learning, Pennsylvania, 7–8, 61, 62

University of St. Thomas, Houston, Texas, 184

University of Tennessee College of Dentistry, 5, 32–34, 50, 51, 97

University of Texas Dental Branch: and Anderson Foundation, 72, 79, 109, 131; Birath as auditor, 84; black students, 133; budgets (1945), 84–85; building for (1940s to 1950s), 93, 108, 109, 130–31, *157;* dental prosthetics, 120; Elliott as dean of, 3, 16, 83–84, 95, 130–31, 134; Elliott honored, 4; Elliott's imaginary walk through (1976), 200; Elliott's portrait, 192; female students, 83; "Medical Horizons" (television, 1956), 156; Olson as dean of, 3; outpatient clinic and Bertner, 110; proposal, 16; Scherer bequest to, 127;

"Television Facilities" and dental viewing, 186–87; Texas Dental College closure (1943), 72, 74, 83–84; and Texas Dental College origins, 5–6, 8, 46–47, 51–52, 66, 69; Texas state legislature lobbying (1940s and 1950s), 13, 16–17, 66–67, 69–71, 76–78, 111–13, 115–19, 126–27; TMC dedication of, 90

University of Texas Medical Branch (UTMB), Galveston: cancer clinic proposal, 12; dental school proposal (1927–31), 44–48; Elliott as stomatology lecturer, 10, 67, 73–74; Elliott seeks university affiliation for Texas Dental College, 5, 6; establishment in Galveston (1890), 38; Hogg's land offer to, 17; Houston move considered (1943), 79, 80–81; leadership conflict, 8–13, 73–75, 77; on probation (1942), 13; Texas state legislature, Spies budget request, 14–15, 66–70, 73

University of Texas (UT): Cancer Foundation, 93, 119, 156, 200; cancer hospital legislation and funding (1941), 13, 14–16, 17, 67–68, 69; chancellorship creation, 118; Development Board, 91–92, 194; Elliott as VP, 95; Graduate School of Biomedical Science, 125, 163; Health Science Center at Houston, 199; Johnson Foundation, 200–201; land deed restriction issues, 105–6; leadership conflict at, 8, 10–13, 77; Medical School, Houston, 90, 132, 136–37, 199; Postgraduate Medical School, 90, 162–63, 181, 191; promotion within TMC, 91–92; School of Nursing, 167–68; School of Public Health, 90, 104–105, 110; Southwestern Medical School, Dallas,

168; Texas Dental College university affiliation sought, 5–6, 8, 46–47, 51–52, 66, 69; Texas Exes (UT alumni), 92–93, 100, 168–69; TMC dedication, 90–91; UT-{\~h}TMC vision brochure, 92–93. *See also* M. D. Anderson Cancer Center
UT. *See* University of Texas (UT)
utilities, TMC, 93, 102, 193
UTMB. *See* University of Texas Medical Branch (UTMB), Galveston

Vateression, L. B., 120
Verheyden, Clyde, 169–70, 182
Veterans Administration Hospital, Houston, 91, 93, 97, 113, 125, 127, 181
Veterans Administration Hospital, San Antonio, 159–60
Villaverde, Christofo and Marquesa de, 146
Voyle, Claude, 129

Wainerdi, Richard E., 206, 207, 208
Walter, M. E., 116
Washington, D.C., Georgetown University, 34
Washington Sun, 96–97
Washington University, 89
Webb, Harry, 111
Weinert, H. H., 85
Weisbrodt, R. H., 46–47
Weiss, Harry C., 129

Weiss Memorial Chapel, 129
Welch, Louis, 155
Wellensiek, Ellen, 83
West, Wesley W., 122
Weston, T. W., 177
White, Leon, 92, 93
White, Paul Dudley, 146
White, William R., 106
Whittington, Mr. and Mrs. Horace, 117
Wilburn, Gene, 166–67, 172, 173–75
Wilkins, Horace M., 16, 18, 68, 86, 141
Williams, Dr. (Texas Dental College faculty), 42
Williams, Georgianna, 56
Williams, O'Bannion, 161, 185
Wilson, George, 53
Wilson, L. R., 11
Wilson, Logan, 148, 154
Winchell, Walter, 128
Wolters, Jacob, 47
Woodley Petroleum Company, 92
Woodward, Dudley Jr., 85, 100, 118
World War I, 29–30
World War II, 15–18, 71–75, 86–87
Wortham, Gus, 116, 166
Wright, Elva, 53
Wright, Geneva Ann, 130
Wright, Theon, 148
Wynn, Percy, 35

YMCA, 106, 184